T0185899

Writing Winning Proposals
for Nurses and
Health Care Professionals

Sandra G. Funk, PhD, FAAN, is a professor emerita of the School of Nursing at the University of North Carolina at Chapel Hill. She has taught research methods, statistics, and grant writing to master's and doctoral students, postdoctoral fellows, visiting scholars, and faculty, and co-teaches with Elizabeth M. Tornquist a program on grant writing. As associate dean for Research and director of the Research Support Center for many years, Dr. Funk led the school's research mission and mentored faculty on design, measurement, proposal development, and research management. She also consults with other universities in these areas. She has served as principal investigator or co-investigator on over $6 million in research funding and served as a reviewer for the National Institutes of Health and other federal agencies for over a decade. Her research interests, grants, and publications, which number over 100, focus on various aspects of applied measurement and research utilization and facilitation.

Elizabeth M. Tornquist, MA, FAAN, has been a faculty member of the Schools of Nursing and Public Health at the University of North Carolina at Chapel Hill and is currently a visiting lecturer at the College of Nursing, University of Arkansas for Medical Sciences. She has taught scientific writing for nearly 40 years and has conducted numerous workshops for university faculty, health care clinicians, and scientists in industry on writing grant proposals, research and technical reports, and articles for publication. She is nationally known as an editor and has helped scientists from many disciplines write fundable grant proposals and publishable articles. In addition, she has authored two books and dozens of articles, and she co-edited three books in addition to those written with Dr. Funk.

Together, Dr. Funk and Ms. Tornquist have taught proposal writing courses and grant-writing institutes; been awarded grants from the National Institutes of Health, the Division of Nursing, and the Agency for Healthcare Research and Quality; developed a research utilization model; published a dozen refereed articles and edited six books (five of which were honored with AJN Book of the Year awards and two of which were republished in other languages).

Writing Winning Proposals
for Nurses and
Health Care Professionals

Sandra G. Funk, PhD, FAAN

Elizabeth M. Tornquist, MA, FAAN

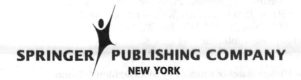

SPRINGER PUBLISHING COMPANY
NEW YORK

Copyright © 2016 Springer Publishing Company, LLC

All rights reserved.

No part of this publication may be reproduced, stored in a retrieval system, or transmitted in any form or by any means, electronic, mechanical, photocopying, recording, or otherwise, without the prior permission of Springer Publishing Company, LLC, or authorization through payment of the appropriate fees to the Copyright Clearance Center, Inc., 222 Rosewood Drive, Danvers, MA 01923, 978-750-8400, fax 978-646-8600, info@copyright.com or on the Web at www.copyright.com.

Springer Publishing Company, LLC
11 West 42nd Street
New York, NY 10036
www.springerpub.com

Acquisitions Editor: Joseph Morita
Composition: Graphic World

ISBN: 978-0-8261-2272-8
e-book ISBN: 978-0-8261-2273-5

15 16 17 18 / 5 4 3 2 1

The author and the publisher of this Work have made every effort to use sources believed to be reliable to provide information that is accurate and compatible with the standards generally accepted at the time of publication. Because medical science is continually advancing, our knowledge base continues to expand. Therefore, as new information becomes available, changes in procedures become necessary. We recommend that the reader always consult current research and specific institutional policies before performing any clinical procedure. The author and publisher shall not be liable for any special, consequential, or exemplary damages resulting, in whole or in part, from the readers' use of, or reliance on, the information contained in this book. The publisher has no responsibility for the persistence or accuracy of URLs for external or third-party Internet websites referred to in this publication and does not guarantee that any content on such websites is, or will remain, accurate or appropriate.

Library of Congress Cataloging-in-Publication Data
Funk, Sandra G., author.
  Writing winning proposals for nurses and health care professionals / Sandra G. Funk, Elizabeth M. Tornquist.
    p. ; cm.
  ISBN 978-0-8261-2272-8—ISBN 978-0-8261-2273-5 (e-book)
  I. Tornquist, Elizabeth M., 1933- , author. II. Title.
  [DNLM: 1. Medical Writing—Nurses' Instruction. 2. Research Design—Nurses' Instruction. WZ 345]
  R119
  808.06′661--dc23
                                2015010373

Special discounts on bulk quantities of our books are available to corporations, professional associations, pharmaceutical companies, health care organizations, and other qualifying groups. If you are interested in a custom book, including chapters from more than one of our titles, we can provide that service as well.

For details, please contact:
Special Sales Department, Springer Publishing Company, LLC
11 West 42nd Street, 15th Floor, New York, NY 10036-8002
Phone: 877-687-7476 or 212-431-4370; Fax: 212-941-7842
E-mail: sales@springerpub.com

Printed in the United States of America by McNaughton & Gunn.

CONTENTS

PREFACE

Whether you are evaluating a new solution to a health problem or trying to move a solution into practice; whether you are interested in training health professionals to work more effectively; or whether you want to show professionals how to implement effective solutions, you must know how to write a successful proposal. And you need to do that throughout your career. This book is designed to help nurses and other health professionals develop compelling proposals for PhD dissertations; National Institutes of Health (NIH) research grants, fellowships, and career development awards; and proposals for education, translation, evidence-based practice, and demonstration projects, including those for the Doctor of Nursing Practice (DNP) capstone project.

Our focus is on giving readers the tools to present the work they are proposing with clarity and conviction—and to show others its importance and potential. This focus comes out of our many years of offering workshops and courses on proposal writing, and editing zillions of proposals. In all those years we have found that students and new investigators often want to do more than can be done in one project and they must learn to think about what's possible, and condense and clarify. At the same time, seasoned investigators sometimes want to just tweak what they have already done, and they must learn to expand. We have also found that investigators often don't understand that a proposal needs to be written over and over again, not put together in one shot and sent off. Therefore, throughout the book we emphasize the importance of thinking, thinking, and thinking; revising and editing; and always asking others for suggestions.

Essentially, our approach is designed to help people think through what they want to do and describe it clearly and succinctly for others. This is the sort of book that nearly all graduate students and young faculty members need in order to build their careers. It also will be useful to practitioners who are interested in developing evidence-based practice. The book can be helpful not only to students but also to their instructors who often struggle with teaching methods while also trying to teach writing about methods. This is not a research-methods text but a book about writing proposals; it can be used as a supplement to research-methods texts in master's level, DNP, and PhD research courses and doctoral seminars.

In Section I: Preparing a Proposal, which we recommend to all readers, we take you through all the parts of developing a proposal, selecting a problem; showing the significance of the problem; describing the work already done on the problem and the need for further work on the problem or its solution; describing your preliminary work, when relevant; and detailing your design and methods. Our aim is to help you think through, organize, and present your ideas, and we include worksheets to aid you in taking the general information we provide and adapting it to your particular project.

In Section II: Types of Proposals, we offer innovative ideas for writing a dissertation proposal or a proposal for a DNP project or other type of evidence-based practice project. Since older models of writing PhD dissertation proposals are not useful when one is seeking funding or real-world approval for evidence-based practice projects, we suggest a more streamlined model for writing PhD or DNP proposals. We provide detailed instructions on how to synthesize relevant literature to make a concise argument for a study and give examples to serve as templates. Then we suggest ways to present methods that are doable and can be carried out in less than a lifetime.

In describing proposals for NIH funding, we give detailed instructions on what content to include and how to organize the Specific Aims section (which is perhaps the most important section of the proposal and is often poorly done), and we provide similar details on writing the Significance, Innovation, and Approach sections. This chapter (Chapter 5) contains in-depth information on writing about the research design and methods. In the chapters on fellowship and career development proposals, we provide clear instructions for developing and presenting your training plan in addition to describing your research plan. And in the educational training grant proposal chapter (Chapter 9), we help you understand what needs to be included in such a proposal, and how to organize and format the information.

In the last two sections, which will be useful to all readers, we offer guidance in composing a title and abstract, preparing the additional materials needed for a proposal, and developing a budget. We also address the processes of writing proposals, submitting a grant proposal, the review, and a possible resubmission.

In sum, over many years we have found that our suggestions have helped people write winning proposals. Thus, for all those who want to change the world, we recommend that you use this book as a guide to proposing change throughout your career.

Sandra G. Funk
Elizabeth M. Tornquist

SECTION I: PREPARING A PROPOSAL

ONE

INTRODUCTION

The purpose of this book is to explain how to write proposals. Unlike most guidelines and similar books, we primarily discuss how you get to the final product rather than what it should look like once you get there (because different proposals "look" different). How do you work with all the literature that is out there to make a concise and coherent argument for your study? What aspects of designing and operationalizing your study should you be thinking about and presenting in the proposal? What do you say about yourself when such information is requested? We tell you. This is not a research methods or statistics book, so be sure to take the courses you need to prepare yourself for what you are hoping to do; this book supplements those courses and your experiences, building on what you have learned.

YOUR GOALS

Your immediate goal in writing a proposal is either to meet a requirement for graduation or to seek funding for your project. Both are important goals, but don't stop there. You also want to use the experience to enhance your credentials—the degree you obtain, the money you are awarded, and the project you conduct all give you opportunities to enhance your résumé (biosketch). The learning itself might not show up on the résumé (e.g, learning to work with others on a project, learning a method or technique, learning an analytic approach) but they can be part and parcel of things that you can put on your résumé: things such as getting the degree, successfully competing for funds, making presentations, and writing papers for publication. So don't only write the proposal. Follow up by doing the proposed project and then writing articles, making presentations and, of course, competing for additional funding to extend the work.

Also use what you propose to do to build the science upon which your project is based. Perhaps no one has applied the intervention you are studying to a particular minority group and you are going to do so. Perhaps there is no pain measurement tool for the demented patient, and you are going to develop one. Perhaps no one has examined ways to help rural patients with diabetes learn about their illness and you are going to evaluate a new approach to meet this need. The degree or funding you receive is designed to enable you to make contributions to the science that will move it forward.

This will also enhance practice, because in the health sciences, the ultimate goal is to help people thrive—to live healthy lives, cope with chronic illness, survive hospitalization without additional illness or re-hospitalization, and so forth. Your goal might be to improve the training of health professionals either while in school or once they are in practice, or perhaps you want to help organize the care that is provided by health professionals in better ways. Whatever your goal, be sure to share your outcomes with the intended population, for only then will your work have the impact you desire.

Remember also that in addition to general goals described previously, some funding opportunities are designed to meet specific goals. For example, the National Institutes of Health's (NIH) Academic Research Enhancement Award (AREA [R15]) is designed to stimulate research in institutions that are less research intensive. The NIH is interested in funding small projects in which students can be involved and get excited about research. With an R15, you become the trainer of others. So in addition to your personal goals and goals to extend the science, there may be other goals you need to keep in mind.

Funding Trajectories

If you are seeking funding, what sort of funding trajectory might be right for you? Everyone differs, but if you are just starting out, you might want to consider fellowships during your predoctoral or postdoctoral studies, or training opportunities as you transition to your next role (e.g., as a faculty member). Why? Because usually these funding opportunities provide support for you and also help to cover insurance, tuition and fees, and minor research expenses. While they tend not to be large amounts, they do support you during a critical time in your development. Another option is small grants that can help in covering some research expenses (some even help pay your salary and insurance). Some people move from a predoctoral fellowship to a postdoctoral fellowship to a training grant to small grants and then on to larger funding—this can be an excellent trajectory for those who need training and wish to do foundational research. Whether you opt for one, some, or all of these funding possibilities, they allow you to show that you can successfully compete for funding, you can manage funds and conduct a project, and you can move through to publication. They also allow you to conduct pilot or preliminary work in order to develop interventions or measures, determine the feasibility of your intervention or research methods, or obtain preliminary estimates of efficacy or estimate effect sizes.

From these types of projects, some people move on to exploratory or developmental projects that will allow them to finish the preliminary work they need to accomplish before conducting definitive studies. Perhaps your fellowship, training, and/or small grant funding enabled you to collect data that guided your development and feasibility testing of an intervention but didn't allow you to obtain preliminary estimates to support its potential efficacy; the developmental/exploratory project might enable you to do this.

After these earlier funded projects, we hope you will move on to larger funding to conduct more definitive studies. Such funding will allow you to support a team of investigators and staff to conduct your project with a larger sample over multiple years. While earlier funding might have enabled you to develop an intervention or measures and obtain preliminary estimates of efficacy, larger funding should be used to test hypotheses about the efficacy of the intervention (or perhaps, subsequently, to determine its effectiveness when put into practice). These larger studies might enable you to explore mediators, moderators, tailoring, and all sorts of additional questions that you could not explore with the smaller samples of the preliminary work. You want a lifetime of funding so you can continue contributing to the science that undergirds practice.

Finding Funding

There are lots and lots of funding opportunities out there. Where and how do you look for ones that might be right for you? Fortunately, today, most of the opportunities are available on the Internet and any search engine you use can probably find them. There are so many opportunities that organizations have been established just to help sift through them (see, e.g., the Community of Science and the Foundation Center listings in Table 1.1). Your institution may have an office that is designed to help you identify funding sources. They might focus on all types of funding or have people with expertise in particular types of proposals: for example, predoctoral or postdoctoral fellowships, training grants, educational grants, or research grants. Be sure to use the resources at your disposal.

Do not ignore intramural funding that might be available from your institution. Many institutions have competitive programs for all types of funding ranging from a variety of doctoral fellowships to travel awards,

TABLE 1.1 Links to a Selection of Funding and Agency Websites

Funding Databases
Community of Science (via ProQuest Pivot) (http://www.cos.com)
The Foundation Center (http://foundationcenter.org)

Federal Agencies
Agency for Healthcare Research and Quality (http://www.ahrq.gov)
Centers for Disease Control and Prevention (http://www.cdc.gov)
Health Resources and Services Administration (http://www.hrsa.gov)
National Institutes of Health (http://www.nih.gov)
National Science Foundation (http://www.nsf.gov)

Foundations/Organizations
Alzheimer's Association, The (http://www.alz.org/index.asp)
American Association for Colleges of Nursing (http://www.aacn.nche.edu)
American Association of Critical-Care Nurses (http://www.aacn.org)
American Association of Neuroscience Nurses (http://www.aann.org)
American Cancer Society (http://www.cancer.org)
American Diabetes Association (http://www.diabetes.org)
American Heart Association (http://www.heart.org/HEARTORG)
American Medical Association (http://www.ama-assn.org)
American Nurses Foundation (http://anfonline.org)
American Pain Society (http://www.americanpainsociety.org)
Arthritis Foundation (http://www.arthritis.org)
Cystic Fibrosis Foundation (http://cff.org)
Eastern Nursing Research Society (http://www.enrs-go.org)
The Kellogg Foundation (http://www.wkkf.org)
Midwest Nursing Research Society (http://www.mnrs.org)
National Association of Pediatric Nurse Practitioners Foundation (http://www
    .napnapfoundation.org/home)
Oncology Nursing Society (http://www.ons.org)
Robert Wood Johnson Foundation (http://www.rwjf.org)
Sigma Theta Tau International, Inc. (http://www.nursingsociety.org/default.aspx)
Southern Nursing Research Society (http://www.snrs.org)
Western Institute of Nursing (http://www.winursing.org)
W. T. Grant Foundation (http://wtgrantfoundation.org)

publication grants, small project grants, and so on. Specialty and regional organizations are also active in funding smaller projects, so don't forget to see what your specialty or regional organization has to offer. Foundations and health organizations typically fund projects in their interest areas, which might be obvious from their titles (e.g., the American Cancer Society, the American Diabetes Association, the American Heart Association, the Cystic Fibrosis Foundation) or may require you to learn their current interests (e.g., the Robert Wood Johnson Foundation, the W. T. Grant Foundation). Federal agencies such as the NIH, the Agency for Healthcare Research and Quality (AHRQ), the Centers for Disease Control and Prevention (CDC), and the Health Resources and Services Administration (HRSA) are big funders of health-related research and education. Indeed, even the National Science Foundation (NSF) funds the science that supports many health topics. All of these agencies can be accessed electronically via the links in Table 1.1, and your institution may have experts in writing proposals for the agency and in reviewing their grants, and perhaps even has sample proposals that you can use to guide your writing.

You should also be creative in thinking about possible funding sources. Who funded the project behind the article you like so much? Check the article—most indicate who funded the project. Don't forget mentors and colleagues. Mentors have a wealth of knowledge about their areas of interest and expertise that (with luck) are in the same area in which you are interested. Colleagues might have heard of something about which you have not heard. Conference presenters usually have a slide that indicates funding sources and so on. Be creative; seek funding wherever you can find it.

Learn About the Funder

As soon as you have identified possible funders, you want to learn what you can about them. Their websites usually have a wealth of information about the agency. Read the mission statement to try to find out what they are generally interested in funding, or what they are currently interested in funding. Perhaps they have an annual report or a direct link to prior grants that will tell you what they have funded in the past and the topics covered. Have they funded folks like you, or are all the funds devoted to people from one discipline, or perhaps to people further along in their careers than you, or perhaps in a topic area that is not a fit for what you are interested in? Do not waste your time trying to convince funders that you or your topic *should* be something in which they are interested. You will end up doing a lot of work but, when push comes to shove, you probably won't be funded.

Some agencies, especially the federal ones, are huge and there is more than one mission statement in which you might be interested. For example, the NIH is currently made up of 27 institutes and centers, each of which has its own mission. So while you want to go to the overall NIH website to start your search (see Table 1.1), you'll also want to click on the link that says "Institutes at NIH," view the listing of institutes, and then click on the link for each institute that might be relevant for you. Read that institute's mission statement; for example, if you are particularly interested in alcoholism among elders, you might wish to check out the National Institute on Alcohol Abuse and Alcoholism and the National Institute on Aging, both of which are part of the NIH. Neither may be interested in your particular project, but it would behoove you to check.

Funding Opportunity Announcement (FOA)

When you have found a funding opportunity of interest, it is time to read the entire announcement (in NIH parlance, this is an FOA). First print it, save it, or at least bookmark the link so you can get back to it (or you may never find it again). If you don't print it, write down its identifying information (e.g., number, title, release date). Check to make sure that you have the most recent announcement—you don't want to do a lot of work for something that is no longer current. Then start your reading. You want to read it at least three times: First, skim the highlights to see if you are eligible to apply for the grant (e.g., if you are a DNP student who wants funding for a capstone project, what does it say about your eligibility?). You can save yourself a lot of reading if you first eliminate the grants for which you are not eligible (but you might want to save them if you think you might be eligible in the future, should the opportunity still be available). Then read the entire FOA to get the details and, finally, reread it because you will have missed more than you thought on the second read.

Now that you have fully absorbed the FOA, look for the fit between you and the funding opportunity. Yes, your eligibility is part of this, but "fit" goes beyond that. You also want to be sure that your institution is eligible. For example, some grants are only for less research-intensive institutions, certain states, or minority-serving institutions. Next, make sure the focus (or one or more of the foci, if there are multiple ones in the FOA) is a fit with your focus. It is critical that your topic fit the funding opportunity. If the funder is only interested in, for example, cancer, you are wasting your time if you prepare a proposal for that funder that is not on cancer. Also, be sure to determine what the due date is for the proposal and whether you can meet it (as outlined in Chapter 15, you may need 3 to 6 months to prepare a proposal). And make sure to check the earliest possible start date for the FOA. For example, some grants may have a 9-month review cycle. Is that okay for you? Do you need to be done with your project before then so that you can graduate? Typically the funder cannot change its review cycle, so you may need to move on to another opportunity or perhaps do the project without funding. Check whether the time period covered by the award and the amount that will be funded are appropriate for your project. These may also help you determine whether the opportunity is a fit with your needs.

Next, note who the contact person is for the FOA and make a list of any questions you have. Ask people locally who might know the answers to your questions—perhaps your mentor, team members, consultants, colleagues, chair, or your institution's grants office. What you cannot get answered locally, hold until you get in touch with the contact person at the funding agency.

Contacting the Agency

What if you just don't know whether the agency (or institute) would be interested in receiving your proposal? Even if you are pretty sure that they *are* interested, we'd recommend that you contact the agency (or institute) and talk to someone who is knowledgeable about their funding programs. Before you make the contact, however, get your ducks in a row: learn what you can about the funder and know what you would like to do. Help yourself by writing out what you would like to do, but be concise and make sure your mentor, if you have one, or another person has read what you have written. Why? It is very hard for the person you contact to help you if you ramble on and on about your project. Be clear about where you are in your career, what kind of support you are seeking, and what the topic area is. Usually you can set up a phone conversation with the agency person, but you might want to email her or him your brief summary in advance of the conversation. You may want your mentor, if you have one, the appropriate associate dean or a knowledgeable colleague, to sit in on your conversation.

Your goal for this conversation is to find out whether the particular agency (or institute) is interested in your topic or perhaps a variant of it. Thus, the contact you make can be very useful to you. Take notes and ask questions, but don't try to convince the person that your project is "just right" if she or he really isn't interested. These people can be excellent at guiding you or perhaps shaping your topic into something in which the agency would be interested. That shaping may be important to you. Do not work on a topic about which you are not passionate, for that passion will sustain you in difficult times. But if a minor variation of the main topic is more fundable, and you are also passionate about that, great. If not, say "thank you" and move on.

Read the Proposal Guidelines

How do you know what to write in your proposal? For each type of proposal, there are guidelines. If you are a student preparing a proposal for perhaps a PhD or DNP program, either your school, your mentor, or the chairperson of your dissertation committee or capstone project provides the specifics needed. If you are applying for funding, the agency to which you are submitting tells you exactly what you need to prepare for your proposal. The NIH has done an exceptional job of detailing what they want for each proposal type (typically using the SF424 [R&R] guidelines). The details they provide can guide you in thinking about many different types of grants, so we place a lot of emphasis on the NIH guidelines in this book. Don't ignore them just because you are not submitting to the NIH at the time. Reading the content may be helpful to you as you prepare other grants. But also be sure to read the guidelines for whatever grant program you are applying to. As with the FOA, you will want to read them multiple times, keep them close by, and refer to them often.

AIDS

The Internet is rife with advice on writing proposals for PhD and DNP work, postdoctoral fellowships, traineeships, research and educational projects, and so forth. Use what is helpful to you, but we recommend that you (a) use this book, (b) consider using any help offered by the funder, and (c) use the help available at your institution (or other institutions) from people with experience submitting to, being funded by, and reviewing grants for the agency in which you are interested. The NIH, in particular, offers a lot of advice and help with respect to preparing successful grant proposals. If you go to the main web page at www.nih.gov, you can play around by clicking on links that look interesting or entering terms in the search engine. Clicking on the "Grants and Funding" link on the header takes you to a lot of resources. Once you click on it, on the left side you will see topics such as "Grant Process Overview," "Grant Application Basics," "Types of Grant Programs," and "How to Apply." All of them have very useful information, so explore. However, we offer a tip: Use the back key if you want to get back to the place from whence you came. The NIH's website is *huge* and can be quite intimidating. After you click on "Grants and Funding," in the center of the page you will see a section about the "NIH Guide for Grants and Contracts." Through this guide, which is issued weekly, the NIH announces new FOAs and policy and rule changes. If you click on "Funding Opportunities and Notices" and scroll down, you will even find a listserv to which you can subscribe to receive weekly emails with links to the newest information. On the right side of the "Grants and Funding" page, you will find the very useful "Rock Talk" (which you can sign up for) and "Latest News," as well as other useful links.

Several of the NIH's institutes and centers have developed and posted on their websites useful aids to proposal writing and submission. For example, the Center for Scientific Review (CSR) has wonderful videos and information for applicants and reviewers that are useful to proposal writers. Also take a look at the National Institute of Allergy and Infectious Diseases (NIAID). You will find grant tutorials and sample applications, along with their reviews. Please note, however, that there is a difference between more biologically driven and more behaviorally driven proposals. At the current time, all of the proposals available on NIAID's website are "hard science" proposals, which might be very different from what you would write for a more behaviorally oriented proposal (i.e., the former often has a set of experiments, each of which is presented in its entirety before moving on to the next one; behavioral proposals, on the other hand, follow the logic presented in this book with a more global presentation of the significance and innovation followed by an approach section).

On the HRSA website (www.hrsa.gov), click on "Grants" to see many useful links about application basics and how to apply. Under its "Funding and Grants" link, AHRQ (www.ahrq.gov) also has useful information on application basics. Even foundations provide guidance and advice on how to successfully apply for their grants. For example, the American Heart Association has a document, *Grant Writing Tips,* available on their website (my.americanheart.org/idc/groups/ahamah-public/@wcm/@sop/ @rsch/documents/downloadable/ucm_426709.pdf).

As noted previously, there are lots of resources at your disposal. One of the presentations we like most is the "How to Fail in Grant Writing" article that appeared in *The Chronicle of Higher Education* some years ago (Jacob, 2010). The article is both hilarious and right on track. Don't forget to read the comments people have added; they offer many additional insights into what works and what doesn't for proposals. Use resources such as this if they facilitate your work; also, you may wish to use them as an adjunct to what you read here.

Best of luck!

REFERENCE

Jacob, E., Porter, A., Podos, J., Braun, B., Johnson, N., & Vessey, S. (2010). How to fail in grant writing. *The Chronicle of Higher Education, 57*(16). Retrieved from http://chronicle.com/article/How-to-Fail-in-Grant-Writing/125620

TWO

RATIONALE FOR THE PROPOSED WORK

The structure of proposals differs depending on what you are proposing to do and where you plan to send the proposal for approval or funding. Clearly, it is essential to follow the required format of the agency or institution to which you are submitting. Yet despite differences in format and organization, the rationale for every study, every evidence-based practice project, and every demonstration project has four parts:

1. There is a problem.
2. Some work has been done on the problem.
3. The work has not gone far enough or it has not been done right.
4. Therefore, this study or this project will take the work further or do it right.

These four parts are not usually presented under separate headings; rather, the argument for the study should flow seamlessly from problem to work on the problem to shortcomings to purpose. To develop this argument, you must first review the literature to find what the problem is, what work has been done on the problem, and what has not been done. Then you develop the argument for a new study or an evidence-based practice project using the literature to document your points. Just as with format, deciding what to include in your description of the literature will depend on the kind of proposal you are writing and the audience. The National Institutes of Health (NIH) reviewers are generally well informed about the research and they assume that you, too, are well informed, so you should provide only a quick review of the literature, focusing on the studies you are building on and showing why more work is needed. On the other hand, readers of a PhD proposal and sometimes readers of a DNP capstone project want to know that you are fully informed about the research in your area, so you may need to describe the problem and the work done on the problem in detail—not to inform your readers but to inform readers that you are informed. Thus, in a proposal for the NIH, the discussion of the literature is short and succinct, whereas in a traditional PhD proposal, the review may be lengthy and all inclusive.

Clearly, a review of the literature is essential for any proposal. Unfortunately, there is not much help available for reviewing the literature, beyond information on search engines to use to find the literature. It helps to think of the review as existing in several stages:

1. Conceptualizing the search
2. Identifying the relevant literature
3. Deciding what to read
4. Reading and analyzing the literature
5. Synthesizing the literature to make the case for your study or project

CONCEPTUALIZING THE SEARCH

Conceptualizing the search is a fancy way of saying you first need to decide what you are looking for. To conduct an effective and efficient search, it is essential to be both descriptive and precise. You will already have looked at some general literature on your topic—that is probably how you discovered that this is an important problem for study. Now you want to review the literature that focuses on the particular aspect of the problem you are interested in. For example, if you are interested in chronic obstructive pulmonary disease (COPD), you do not want to go to a search engine and punch in COPD—because the articles will come tumbling out in wheelbarrow loads, and you could spend the rest of your life reading them. Instead, list words that describe the aspect of this overall problem that you intend to study. Will you focus on prevention of disease progression, exercises to improve endurance, exacerbations of COPD, hospitalization experiences, interventions to improve management at home, problems experienced by caregivers, end-of-life care? Your list of words should precisely reflect the focus of your proposed study.

As you develop the list, remember that librarians index journal articles based on words, usually key words in the title and sometimes additional key words supplied by authors and listed under the title or at the bottom of the title page. If you do not use the same words the indexer used, you will not find an article. (This, incidentally, is why authors who use a cute title always follow it with a colon and words indicating what the article is really about.) Thus, it is important to spend some time thinking about the words to use in making a search. And interestingly, that thinking will not only make your literature search more effective and efficient, but it will also make your study focus clearer and more precise. For example, if you are interested in preventing unnecessary hospitalizations for heart failure, thinking about words to use to find causes of unnecessary hospitalizations and existing interventions to prevent these hospitalizations may help you decide whether you want to focus on interventions made directly with the patient, with a family caregiver, or with practitioners who may need to provide more information and support to patients and families.

IDENTIFYING THE RELEVANT LITERATURE

Once you have a list of words, decide what combinations of them to use; then go to the computer and institute the search. There is plenty of information available on how to access PubMed, CINAHL, and so forth, and these sources will provide most of the materials you want. However, in addition to looking at databases, you should always check the reference lists of the articles you retrieve. You may find articles listed that your search did not turn up and you may also see key words in article titles that might be used to expand your search. It is also helpful to ask for "like articles" in databases such as PubMed and to examine the list of studies currently being funded by the NIH to identify work in your area that has not yet been published. Finally, it is useful to collect programs from the conferences you attend: You can e-mail presenters in your area to ask for an abstract or a copy of an article that may be accepted for publication but has not yet appeared. And the more you present and publish your own work, the more you will hear about others' work; that is one way to stay current on what is being done in your area.

It is important to read all the relevant literature; but it is also important not to drown in the literature. "I can't write until I read more" is a frequent refrain, especially among people new to the literature who fear that somehow they will miss the key articles unless they scour the literature and find everything. You are unlikely to miss the key articles; if you do not find them in your searches, you will probably find them in the reference lists of the articles you do find. As we noted earlier, if you check the NIH website and keep programs from conferences, you should be able to identify work that is new and not yet published.

Sometimes the literature in your area is scant. However, it is likely that people somewhere have done something about the problem you are interested in. Of course, it is possible that they have not published. (This occurs most often when interventions have not achieved the expected effects. It is hard to publish those studies though they may be productive failures; i.e., they may provide useful information about what works and what does not work.) However, the relevant work may not be showing up in your search because you have not used the right search terms. It can be helpful to discuss these with a librarian—remember librarians are the people who index articles and they have a keen eye for search terms and key words. If you still do not find anything, even with help, expand the search. If nothing has been done in your discipline, it is always possible that people in other disciplines have done work that bears on the problem or its solution. Sometimes this work will not have been done in health care but in economics, sociology or psychology, and so forth. Therefore, you want to look as broadly as possible.

And in some cases you may need to expand your search beyond the standard databases. For example, if you are studying a recent development in health care, you should probably look at the *New York Times* index, because investigative journalists often have information on developing problems or approaches in health care before they are reported in the scientific literature. The reason for this is that it takes time, often a lot of time, to get articles into the scientific literature, and investigative journalists can move faster. *The New Yorker* and other intellectual magazines also publish thoughtful articles on health care that are often ahead of others. It is useful to read such journals—they will help your thinking as well as your retrieval of relevant materials.

DECIDING WHAT TO READ

Once you have a list of articles, you have to decide which ones to read. Our general advice is to read the most recent work. Science advances based on the latest information, not old ideas. If you have a list of articles published in the past 10 years, you might try first reading articles published in the past 2 years; then, if the literature is thin in your area, read back further. Do not automatically start reading articles published 10 years ago and move forward: Unless you are writing about a historical development, you will waste a lot of time reading information that is outdated.

Sometimes, of course, you need to read older work. For example, you may be interested in theories that were published years ago. If you are interested in Freud's theories, you need to read Freud, who published his work mostly in the early 20th century. (If you reference Freud with a date of 2005, for example, readers will immediately know that you did not read Freud; you read somebody who read him, and you will look bad.) Also, you may want to read the seminal work in your area: When you see author after author referencing a particular study or researcher, that is a sign that the person is important and you probably need to read the work. Finally, sometimes you have to read older articles because there is no recent work in your area. That happens because research topic areas are like clothes or young girls' hairstyles—the fashions change. Some topics, like cancer or cardiovascular disease, never go away, but others come and go. For example, interest in death and dying first surfaced more than 50 years ago with Kübler-Ross's description of the stages of dying. For a few years people in health care were tremendously interested in death and dying. Then interest waned and for a period there was little work on the topic. Dying became a fashionable topic again when hospice was first introduced in this country from England. Over the next few years, there were dozens of articles published on hospice care. Then that interest waned. More recently, the topic of dying has gained favor again, with work on end-of-life care and palliative care. Thus, if you are planning a project in a currently unfashionable area, you may not find much in the literature—but on the other hand, you may also be exploring new territory, which will make your work more easily funded!

Sometimes there is a great deal of literature in your area. If that is the case, you first need to carefully consider whether something more is needed. Are there interventions that have been found effective, and if so, why do you need to develop and test another intervention? For example, the dietary approaches to stop hypertension (DASH) diet, developed to reduce hypertension, has been shown to be effective in helping people lose weight. Why do we need another diet? We might—but what we more likely need is an intervention that helps people follow the DASH diet, not another diet program. Similarly, the Centers for Disease Control and Prevention (CDC) have recommended an intervention that is effective for self-managing diabetes. Why do we need another one? We might; but again, what we need is probably an intervention that helps people do what we already know is effective in managing diabetes. So your review of the literature should help you decide what is needed now, and if your initial ideas need to be changed, this is the time to do that.

By the way, it is important to recognize that you do not review the literature only when you are planning a proposal. Whenever you read, you are reviewing the literature. Therefore, you should never read an article in your area of interest without making a note about it and a complete bibliographic citation. (When you find an article to be useless, be sure to make a note about that, otherwise you are likely to read it again and again, particularly if it has a seductive title.) If you keep good records on what you read even when you are not conducting a systematic review of the literature, you will not have to go searching for an article that you read last year and liked. You will have it in your records. This is how you build your grasp of the literature; over time you will become familiar with most of the work in your area and when you plan a new proposal, you will only have to check the databases to see what has been done in recent months.

READING AND ANALYZING THE LITERATURE

As a researcher or a practitioner interested in evidence-based practice, you need to read a lot of articles reporting research, that is, evidence. Unfortunately, that is not easy. In part this is because research is not always clearly presented and it is therefore difficult to decipher. And you may not have been taught to decipher it efficiently. Some research courses teach students to struggle through every research article from start to finish, then critique the article based on a checklist approach. Does the article have a theoretical framework? If so, check; that is a good article. If not, no check, meaning that is not a good article. But this approach is useless. The questions that matter are: Did the study's theoretical framework make sense? Did it provide a guiding conceptualization for the study? Or was the framework so broad that anything could have fit within it? Did the authors talk about whether it was useful and how?

Similarly, students are often taught to ask the wrong questions about a study sample. Did the study have a big sample? Check, good study. Did it have a small sample? No check, not good study. But suppose the study was examining factors that contribute to ventilator–associated pneumonia in the intensive care unit—how long would it take to get a big sample in such a study? Maybe years. Thus, it is important to think about articles reporting studies in a different way.

One extremely useful approach to writing about research was described by Huth (1999). According to Huth, we read scientific papers not simply to get the answers to questions or the solutions to problems—if we did, we would need only to read a study's abstract, because the abstract usually tells us what the problem was and offers the solution or answer. No, we read to see the critical argument of the study. Every scientific paper makes a critical argument. This argument has four parts: (a) there is a question that needs to be answered or a problem that needs to be solved; (b) there is some evidence for a conclusion about that question or problem; (c) there is a discussion of the credibility of the evidence; and (d) there is a conclusion.

While Huth uses this approach to tell writers how to present their research, we think it is equally useful to look at the critical argument when you read articles reporting research. First, note that the four parts of a critical argument are the same as the four parts of a research article, in a slightly different order. In a research report, everything before the methods section is a description of the issue, question, or problem and why it needed to be studied. The methods section is a description of the credibility of the findings (or evidence): Authors tell you their methods so that you will trust the accuracy and generalizability of what they found. The findings section is the evidence for the conclusion, and the conclusion comes in the final discussion.

If you are looking at the critical argument of a study, the first thing you want to know is what the conclusions are. First, read the title of the article. Some articles, particularly in medical journals, tell you the conclusion of the study straight off: "Drug X Improves Condition Y." That is what the authors concluded from the evidence they found. The titles of articles in nursing and public health journals are not generally that direct. However, if the title is something like this: "The Effectiveness of Intervention X in Improving Condition Y," then clearly the authors think the study provided evidence that their intervention worked (even if at the end they say the sample was too small to generalize the findings to others). If they had not found the intervention effective, the authors would not have titled their article "The Effectiveness of...." If they had found it ineffective they certainly would not have titled it, "The Ineffectiveness of...." When researchers do not find some evidence that their intervention has been useful, they are more likely to use a long title, such as this one: "The Possibility That Factors X and Y May Be Related to the Effect of Intervention A on the Outcomes of Condition Z." A quick rule of thumb is this: The longer the title, the greater the likelihood that findings were inconclusive or mixed.

Thus, the title gives you an initial sense of the authors' conclusions. But then read the abstract, which will tell you what the question or problem was and what the answer was. Sometimes titles are seductive—but when you read the abstract, you discover that the study was not even about the topic suggested by the title. If the article is not on the topic you are interested in, you do not need to waste time reading the article.

Once you have established that this is a relevant article, go to the discussion section to identify the authors' conclusions. These may be spread through several small sections titled Discussion, Implications for Practice, and Conclusions, which often give the same information over and over. Or the conclusions may be presented in one section at the end of the article. Your goal is to find out what these conclusions are.

Sometimes the authors' conclusions are not clear; alas, many researchers end the reports of their studies by saying that their sample was too small or too homogeneous or too geographically restricted to be generalizable to anybody different and nothing can be concluded until more research is done. (That is one reason why many clinicians do not read research. After they have read countless articles describing interventions that seem to be effective and are then told, "For God's sake don't use this," clinicians give up.) Authors always have conclusions, but they may not tell you what these conclusions are because they are afraid someone will criticize them. So if the conclusions are not clear, or there seem to be no useful conclusions, you have to figure them out. Go back to the findings section to see what the conclusions ought to be and then check their credibility by examining the study methods. For example, if the authors found that a program to reduce binge drinking by young men was successful but concluded that their findings were not generalizable because the sample was too small or the study was conducted in only one city, what did the findings actually show? Did binge drinking drop significantly more in the intervention group than in a control or comparison group? Over what period of time? What else happened? Why did the authors think their findings could not be used by others? Was their reasoning good, or was this a knee-jerk response based on conservative views about what can be generalized and what needs more research? In the end, even if the findings are not broadly generalizable, the study may have been conducted in a clinic or community center enough like yours to make the findings useful for you.

When you know what the conclusions are (or should be), if they are not interesting or promising, you may not need to read anything more. If the conclusions appear promising, go back and read the full article to see if the introduction makes clear the reason for the study, and the methods and findings justify the conclusions.

When you read through the study, try to do so efficiently. Note that in biomedical journals the introductory section is getting shorter and shorter, with less and less description of the literature. That is because, like life, reading is going faster. In the Discussion section, authors usually compare their findings to the findings of others, and thus the research closest to that being reported is described near the end of the article. In the past, readers wanted to see nothing in the Discussion section that was not mentioned in the Introduction. Now, readers do not want to hear about the literature both at the beginning and the end of an article—life is too short, so authors only talk generally about the literature at the beginning and discuss the most relevant articles in more detail later. Some nursing journals continue to include a lengthy introductory section, often with several headings: Introduction, Background, Review of the Literature, The Problem, Theoretical Considerations, and so forth. But much of that material is repetitious and you may not need to read it all. You can usually find enough information to decide whether the study is important by reading the Introduction and the last few sentences before the Methods section. If a study seems important, however, you may want to check the authors' use of the literature to see whether their review helps you conceptualize your own approach to the literature.

Next read the Methods and Findings. For example, if the authors concluded that their intervention reduced obesity in school-age children, you want to see whether the findings actually justify this conclusion, which requires you to look at both what the authors did and how it turned out. Did the children who got the intervention lose significantly more weight than a control group who did not receive the intervention? Was the sample big enough to determine that? What if the sample was too small to test the significance of differences between those who received the intervention and those who did not: Did the findings show some trends toward improvement? In what? Did the children consume fewer calories? Exercise more? Show more understanding of what their bodies needed and why? How did the authors measure those? By asking these questions, you can determine whether the conclusions are solid enough to build on, or whether they are weak and, if so, why. This kind of analysis also helps you to determine what needs to be done to ensure that the intervention you are proposing will be effective.

When you are reviewing findings, do not just believe any statistics you see; there is a lot of error out there in the world of study reports. For example, did the authors present the information used to determine the power of the statistical testing? Was the sample size sufficient? Were the variables used to determine the outcomes well measured? Were the researchers testing hypotheses or just data snooping? Were there lots of missing data? Were the data analyzed correctly? (You may want to seek consultation on this if statistics are not a strength of yours.) If multiple tests were done, was the error rate adjusted to account for this?

If lots of data were missing or the final sample size was not adequate, the measurements did not appear to be appropriate, or you felt there were other problems with the analysis, you will give less credence to the findings. However, you may still use them to suggest variables or dimensions that you will evaluate further in your own study.

If this was a qualitative study, you also need to look at methods: Did the authors provide information on the sample, describe the way they collected data (not a textbook explanation but a description of what they actually did) and tell you how they analyzed and categorized the findings? Did the categories match the quotes from participants? If the authors described themes, what did those themes mean?

The next step is documenting what you have read. Be sure to make a complete bibliographic citation for every article—you do not want to be trying to figure out where that note about the effects of bullying on gay adolescents came from when you are completing the proposal. And make a note to indicate what was useful in every article. Perhaps the findings were impressive, or the authors had interesting suggestions for further research in their Discussion section. Or they used an instrument to measure attitudes that could be very helpful in the study you are proposing. Those notes will help you when you go back to articles later. If you do not make such notes, you are likely to forget what mattered in an article and even the article itself (nothing is so forgettable as scientific articles, except possibly detective novels).

When you have completed your systematic review, it is helpful to make a table that summarizes the most important information in key articles. These are generally the articles reporting studies most similar to what you are planning; you will need to show that you are building on these, yet are different. It takes some time to put together such a table, but it can save you time later. For example, if you have concluded that the time covered in a study was too short to provide useful information, when you are writing your proposal, you can check the table to get the data on that; you do not have to keep rereading the article to find it. A table may also be useful if later you decide to write a review article on the literature on your topic.

In putting together the table, it is helpful to use article abstracts to find out what the authors of a study thought was important, though you will often find surprising omissions of crucial information in abstracts; and sometimes instead of giving conclusions, the author will say "conclusions are discussed"—an indication that they may be complicated. In your table always be sure to include not just methods and findings, but also conclusions (Table 2.1).

TABLE 2.1 Possible Format for Table of Literature Read

Author/ Article Title	Purpose	Setting and Sample	Intervention (If Relevant)	Variables/ Measures	Findings	Conclusions	Journal/ Date

SYNTHESIZING THE LITERATURE TO MAKE THE CASE FOR YOUR STUDY OR PROJECT

Critically reading the literature is important in developing the rationale for a study or project, but effectively synthesizing the literature to articulate that rationale is even more important. This is how you show readers that the problem or question you plan to study is important, and that there has been some work on the problem or question but it has not gone far enough or been adequately done.

As you read, always make notes. After you have read the articles, made notes on them, and perhaps put together a table like one described earlier, the next step is to look at your notes and figure out what is there—what the literature amounts to. In his book *The Lives of a Cell: Notes of a Biology Watcher*, Thomas (1974) noted that science advances in the way we put together jigsaw puzzles. The people who begin a new line of research or establish the parameters for new research are the people who put together the outside pieces of the puzzle. Then the rest of us come along and put pieces in the puzzle—I put a piece here and you put a piece there and somebody else puts a piece in after us, until we complete the puzzle. Then we move on to the next puzzle. The literature is what is already in the puzzle, and our task is to look at the literature to see what has been done, then add to it. But alas, there is no picture on the cover of this puzzle. That is not a problem when there are only 20 or so pieces left. By then the picture is clear. But in the early stages of putting a puzzle together, we do not know what the pieces already in the puzzle stand for: That blue piece near the corner could be the sky or the ocean or somebody's skirt. What has the research achieved thus far? And what pieces are still needed to complete the puzzle? What work still needs to be done?

Sometimes people think that the literature will give them the argument for a study or project, if they just read the articles through again—and again—and maybe again. But the articles you read will never give you the argument for your study because they were not written for that purpose. They were written for their own purposes; you have to make your own argument. And you probably have a pretty good sense of that argument by now. The task is to make it clear to others.

This requires synthesizing the literature in a coherent, logical fashion. Unfortunately, few people are taught to synthesize the literature—because it is difficult: difficult to do and difficult to teach. But we have some suggestions for this.

Organize your discussion of the literature using the outline listed at the beginning of this chapter: problem, work done on the problem, shortcomings in the work to date and, finally, purpose of the proposed study or project. Then separate the articles you have examined into groups. But do not group articles by subject—for example, elderly women, depression, fatigue, heart attack—because this kind of grouping will not help you synthesize the literature into an argument for your study. Instead, group together general review articles on the problem, individual studies that provide key data on the particular aspect of the problem you will work on, articles describing various interventions for the problem (if you plan an intervention), and finally, the studies closest to what you plan. These studies are most important because they show what you are building on; after describing those studies, you must show how your work differs from that work—takes it further or does it more adequately. Therefore, discuss these studies last and give them the most attention. (Note that some articles may provide information on the problem and describe a solution to the problem, so they belong in both groups.)

The Problem

Always start with the problem. In health care studies or projects, the problem is either a problem in health or a problem in health care. For example, the fact that one out of every eight or nine women in the United States will have breast cancer is a problem in health. So is the fact that approximately one out of ten people in this country will have diabetes. But the fact that we still have difficulty controlling pain is a problem in health care, as is the fact that many elderly hospitalized patients are not routinely assessed for delirium.

Most people planning to conduct a study or a project know what the problem is. That is what led them to think about a study or project. However, sometimes they forget to tell readers what that problem is, or they do not state the problem directly, or they do not identify the aspect of the problem they will focus on, and then readers have no idea why their particular study or project is needed. Therefore, it is essential to begin your proposal by first telling readers what problem you are addressing. If the problem is big—for example, the high prevalence of asthma in children, especially low-income children, you are unlikely to be planning a study or project to solve the whole problem. Rather, you may plan to address a part of the problem or a particular aspect of it, or you may plan an intervention to address a particular aspect of the problem or a particular group with the problem.

Though you may not plan to address the whole problem, always begin by showing its importance. A problem is important for one of three reasons. Though not very serious, it is widespread, like the common cold. Or though not common, it is very serious, like Huntington's chorea. Or it is both common and serious, like HIV infection. You establish the importance of a problem by providing evidence from the literature—figures on its prevalence, its consequences, its costs. Do not, however, begin with a generalization such as "Asthma in children is a serious public health problem." Such general statements are like warm-up pitches—they are useful in helping you to begin but are not part of the game, so get rid of them.

Go straight to the data: "In the United States, the prevalence of asthma is high among children [give the figures], with serious adverse consequences [name them and provide references]." You want to show the importance of the problem, not just tell it—the key throughout is to show, not tell.

The better known the problem, however, the less you have to say about it. For example, if you plan to study risk for diabetes in a particular group, the people who review your proposal will all know that diabetes is a major problem in the United States; you need to give the figures on prevalence and consequences, but you do not need to provide a long description of the disease in order to convince readers that diabetes is widespread and leads to major complications. Similarly, everyone knows that HIV is a serious problem; we do not have to be told that, readers just need the latest figures. However, if you are working on a rare cancer that many people have not even heard of, you will need to show why it is important and why there is a need to do something about it, and that may take a good deal more documentation than you can give in a sentence or two.

One caution: If you have a great deal of information about a problem, it is tempting to tell readers all about it, even if they do not need the information. This is a particular problem for beginning researchers: Sometimes they do not realize that while they are just discovering the depth and breadth of some problem, other people already know about it. Also, after going to all that trouble to read dozens of articles on the problem, it is hard to just put the literature aside; however, you can save it for a review paper or a book chapter on the topic. Here it will waste your space and annoy readers.

After describing the overall problem, note the aspect of the problem you will address and its importance, or note the importance of the problem for a particular population or the need for a solution to the problem. Sometimes, if the overall problem is extremely well known, such as diabetes, you may go straight to the aspect you are going to study, say, foot ulcers in those with diabetes. Generally, however, you first say something about the big problem. For example, you may plan to examine factors that contribute to asthma in children or disparities in the prevalence of asthma, or parents' need for information or resources to manage the disease. Or you may plan to intervene to help parents better manage children's symptoms at home. First, as noted earlier, you give the prevalence of asthma in children, then move on to your particular focus.

If the big problem is hypertension, you may plan to examine factors involved in the early development of hypertension in young African American men, or barriers to medication adherence among this group. Briefly note the prevalence of hypertension, then point out the importance of the particular issues you will address and provide evidence from the literature to support that importance. You may need to briefly describe individual studies on this aspect of the problem, rather than just giving a couple of general sentences, but that will depend on how well this aspect of the problem is known, and you will figure that out from reading the literature.

The Work Done on the Problem

Making the case for the importance of the problem is usually not very difficult; describing what has been done on the problem is more challenging. To do so, you review the literature describing the problem and what has been done about it (rarely is this section called Review of the Literature other than in traditional dissertation proposals and perhaps DNP capstone project proposals). In describing the literature, there is always a question about where you should describe theoretical work on the problem. If there has been significant theoretical work in developing knowledge of the problem or in suggesting solutions, and this work has served as a foundation for studies done on the problem, you may want to include this theoretical work early in the discussion of the literature, along with articles describing the general problem or general solutions—before you describe particular studies, because it provides the basis for those studies. However, if the theoretical work does not serve as the basis for general work on the problem but instead will guide your study by providing a framework for conceptualizing the problem and a possible solution to the problem, then it is more logical to describe the theoretical work after describing other work on the problem. The most appropriate place is in the section on your conceptual framework. Otherwise you are likely to end up describing theory twice—both in the review of the literature and the conceptual framework sections. This is a judgment call, however; try it in both sections and see what works best.

The section on work done on the problem presents your understanding of the research done to date. If you plan to investigate some aspect of the problem of diabetes that few people have explored—for example, the experiences of adolescents newly diagnosed with type 2 diabetes—you will have noted the importance of diabetes earlier and pointed out that type 2 diabetes is increasing among the young. Here you need to describe the findings of studies that looked at adolescents. Do not, however, describe the study methods unless these are related to what you plan. This review should give readers a good sense of what is already known, not a summary of every study you have read. Begin with the more general studies, then, as noted earlier, move to the studies that are closest to what you plan to do.

If you are proposing to examine a problem—for example, posttraumatic stress disorder (PTSD) in a group that has not been included in most earlier studies, such as children and adolescents who have come to this country from war zones—first briefly describe the work that has been done on refugee populations with PTSD, then review in more detail any studies about children and adolescents experiencing this syndrome or showing problems that might suggest PTSD. Again, focus on the findings of the studies, not their methods. If the literature suggests that PTSD may be common in these children, then it will be important to find out whether that is the case so that something can be done about it.

If you are proposing a new intervention for a particular group, you need to focus on the interventions that have already been tested with this group and their effects on the problem. For example, if your interest is in arm movements of persons who have suffered a stroke, in the section describing the problem you will have noted that these people have difficulty with arm movements. If you are proposing to test a new approach to help them expand their reaching ability, first describe what has already been done to improve their capacity. Later you will need to note the shortcomings of these interventions and show why a new approach may have more potential for success.

Sometimes numerous interventions for a particular problem have been tried, with more or less success. For example, there have been many interventions designed to help school children lose weight. However, the prevalence of overweight and obesity in this group is not going down substantially. First describe the overall work on interventions, then describe the interventions closest to the approach you are planning and their outcomes. You want to give readers a clear sense of what has been achieved. Then point to possible reasons for lack of effectiveness in the work done to date, to provide a basis for suggesting that your intervention has greater potential than the others.

If nothing has been published in your area, it is tempting to conclude that nothing has been done, but as noted earlier, that is almost never the case. Something has always been done; perhaps nothing has been done in your discipline, but something that bears on the problem or the solution has been done by someone. There is hardly anything new under the sun. We always start from something, not nothing. The something may be clear or it may be difficult to find.

Thus, your relationship to the literature may be of two types—linear or many branched. The relationship is linear when the research to date has developed in a straight line, but has not gone far enough, or has not been done in a way that actually solves the problem. In this case, what you plan to do is extend the line further—to a different population, a different problem, or a different age group, or you plan to try a different intervention. For example, a great deal of research has shown that hepatitis C contributes to the development of liver cancer. But perhaps you are interested in an Asian population that appears to have a high incidence of hepatitis C and liver cancer but no one has actually studied this population. In such a case, simply describe what has been done to date and point out that your target group has not been studied, or existing interventions have not been tried with them. Thus, you take a straightforward approach to the literature. Group A has been done, B has been done, C has been done and all this research is convincing. However, group D has not yet been studied but must be because the people in this group are in need.

Similarly, the research may have developed in a linear fashion but the methods of the latest studies have not been adequate or appropriate to solve the problem. For example, research has clearly shown the enormity of the problem of HIV infection among young African Americans. Moreover, research has shown the utility of testing and preventive behaviors like condom use. However, the interventions tested to date have not been effective in reaching some of the people most at risk and helping them change their behaviors, and thus infections continue to increase in this group. Therefore, a new intervention is needed. Again, you take a straightforward approach to the literature. Approach A has been done, B has been done, and C has been done but C has not been effective so we need to try D, a new approach that has greater potential to succeed.

Whether you are taking the research further or taking an approach that may be more effective than the work to date, you have a relatively simple relationship to the literature: You are advancing in a straight line. In other cases, however, the literature you are using is like the many branches of a tree. There is no work that leads directly to what you are planning. There is some useful information in one article and some in another article, but the information may come from the work of other disciplines or the work on an entirely different problem, and it may not easily add up to an argument for what you are planning. In this case, you have to extrapolate findings from various studies and show how these can be interpreted to make the case for your work. Making such a case is far more difficult than making a linear case, because to show how work in other areas provides a foundation for what you plan, you need to not only summarize the studies but also explain their applicability to your proposed work.

First, document the existence of the problem (with appropriate references) and, next, point out that no reported work is directly related to the work you are proposing because no one has examined the problem or no one has taken the approach you are planning. Then say that there is a basis for your plans from the work in other fields or with other problems or with other groups. Next, briefly summarize the studies on the other problems or groups, focusing on findings. In describing the studies, point out the similarities to your problem or approach and note the potential applicability of this other work. Although dealing with the literature in this way is difficult, because there is little or nothing in your particular area and you have to reach afield, your proposed study may also be newer, more innovative, and thus more interesting than a study that simply takes established research a step further.

Shortcomings in the Work Done to Date

The key to justifying a new study is showing that either the work to date has not gone far enough or it has not been done right. However, after you have pointed out the contributions that others have made, you cannot simply say, "There is a gap in what is known." What gap? Sometimes there is a gap that does not need to be filled, so do not just have a knee-jerk reaction to gaps. This sort of vague buzzword is not helpful. You must clearly show that earlier work has not focused on problems that are important for study or has not targeted vulnerable groups, or earlier interventions have not been effective or effective enough. Perhaps, studies have been done with some people but not with others, even though these unstudied people are a major or growing proportion of the population, or a group that desperately needs interventions. For example, as we all know, in the past, studies of cardiovascular disease focused on White, mostly middle-age men; heart problems in women and African Americans were ignored though the prevalence of heart disease is higher in African Americans than in Whites, and among older Americans it is higher among women than among men. Numerous recent studies have therefore focused on these groups, and have found significant differences from White middle-age men, providing a foundation for ongoing development of interventions for these groups.

Perhaps an intervention or approach has been found effective with participants who have a particular disease, but the approach has not been tried with another group that has the disease. However, if you plan to use an approach that has been shown to be effective, you must be clear about why a new test is needed. You cannot tweak an intervention just a little for a new group—if an intervention simply needs a little tweaking, do that and put it into practice: You do not need funding for a new study. Show why new work is needed. Perhaps the population is so different that you cannot implement the intervention as it exists but must adapt it to the new group. For example, you may need to adapt a proven self-management intervention for diabetes to make it work with Hispanic patients with low health literacy. Or perhaps the intervention needs to be adapted in order to be widely usable in practice. For example, an intensive intervention to reduce depression in pregnant women may need to be adapted for use with low-income women who receive care in a health department.

Perhaps interventions developed to solve a problem have had only limited success. If so, it is important to explain why earlier efforts have failed. Perhaps others did not solve the problem because their methods were not the best way to approach the problem. To illustrate, in the past, health care providers often seemed convinced that all they needed to do was tell people how they should behave, based on the research, and then people would do what was good for them. If people were told about the effectiveness of the DASH diet for losing weight, they would immediately stop eating fried bacon and switch to broccoli and cauliflower. If they were told they should cut down on their drinking, they would do so. These interventions did not take into account the fact that people may not want to behave differently and they will perversely do what they want to do. Also, most of us live with a certain amount of inertia: Habits die hard and we tend to do what we have always done, so getting us to change is a major challenge. Finally, often interventions have not factored in the difficulties of people's lives or the stresses they face. For example, some studies of interventions to increase exercise in older, low-income women did not take into account the fact that many live in unsafe neighborhoods where walking outside is dangerous and there are no other places to exercise. Or interventions to get people to take their medicine did not consider that when people do not have enough money, they may choose to buy food for their children rather than buying medications for themselves. Thus, the interventions were doomed to failure. As a result, recent interventions have often tried to take into account what are called social determinants of health, or the world in which people live, and help people deal with their lives and the situations they are in.

If you are planning to try a new and different intervention to change people's behavior, you must be clear about the shortcomings of other interventions. This is where you provide some detail about these interventions and the methods used to test them. However, focus on explanations for lack of success; do not summarize overall methods. And you may be able to combine studies. For example, you might note that several studies have tested group interventions for Hispanics with diabetes, but none have included family members in the groups, and their failure to take into account the family focus of the Hispanic culture may explain their lack of effectiveness in helping participants control their diabetes. Then reference all the studies; you do not need to describe each one of them.

If you are planning to use new technology—perhaps the newest smartphone—to engage a particular group of people in making change (eating better, exercising more, or avoiding risky sex), give only a brief description of the many interventions that have been shown to help people make that change, if they will but follow them. Then describe in more detail the studies that have tested interventions with this particular group and report their methods and their successes. Next point out the shortcomings of these interventions. Did they have only short-term effects? Were they resource-intensive? Did they require people to come to meetings? Then describe any studies that have used the new technology and indicate why and how the technology is effective or appears likely to be effective with the group you will study. Finally, state why another study is needed with this technology. It may be that no interventions have used the technology for this problem or this group, though studies have used it for other problems or groups and have provided evidence of its potential for success. If so, point out that the technology has not been used with your problem or group and indicate why a test of this is needed. If there have been studies of the use of the technology with this group, you must indicate the ways in which your intervention differs.

In sum, you must show two things: You are building on the work that has already been done, and you are doing something that has not been done but needs to be done—you are not simply repeating others' work. Your description must clearly show that your approach differs from the efforts to date and you are not simply going to repeat the mistakes you have just criticized—or do something that looks even less likely to succeed. Otherwise readers will think this person is simply doing what has already been done, and wonder why it will succeed this time when other interventions have failed.

You cannot, for example, say that the interventions to date have been less than successful because they focused only on individuals although the problem is really a family problem, and then propose to also focus only on individuals. Also you cannot say we are unable to draw any conclusions about the efficacy of an intervention because the studies to date have not assessed effects over a long enough period of time, and then say you plan to assess effects over the same short period of time.

One caveat here: Replication is the essence of science. If you have found an effective intervention, you may want to replicate it. Indeed, if an experiment cannot be repeated, or an intervention cannot be found effective more than once, then we cannot conclude anything from the work. Yet, it is difficult to get funding for a straightforward replication. Therefore, if you plan to replicate an intervention it is wise to try the intervention with another group or another problem.

Finally, be careful not to denigrate the work you are building on. It is not useful to say that researchers to date have failed because they did not understand reality; instead, you want to say that prior researchers have made extremely useful contributions in studying the problem or in developing and testing interventions for the problem, but given the complexities of people's lives or the difficulties of this problem, or the changing demographics of our society, more is now needed. (This is important not only because it is scientifically reasonable but also because it is politically sound: The people who review your proposal for funding may well be the people who tested those earlier interventions—you want to be grateful to them.)

The final part of the argument for your study is this: Although work has been done on this important problem, the work is less than adequate or remains unfinished and therefore your purpose is to take it further or do it right. So conclude this section of the proposal by stating or restating your study's purpose.

DEVELOPING A CONCEPTUAL FRAMEWORK

Many research proposals include a description and often a drawing of the conceptualization or framework to be used to guide the study and show its potential for success. This framework should be described after the argument for the study has been made. The best place for it is immediately following the purpose statement. Essentially you say, "Here is what our purpose is and here is how we are conceptualizing the study to achieve that purpose."

However, it is important to recognize that not every study requires a conceptual framework. The more physiological the proposed study, the less likely it is to include a conceptual framework—the scientific reasoning behind aims, hypotheses or questions is, in fact, the conceptual basis for the study. The more behavioral the work, the more likely it is to include a conceptual framework and to draw on labeled theory. For example, for many years researchers have used the Transtheoretical Model of Change (Prochaska & DiClemente, 1982) as a framework for tailoring interventions to people whose behaviors they are trying to change. First used in efforts to reduce smoking, this model basically says that a one-size intervention does not work for all, just as a one-size shirt or dress does not fit everyone. If a person is ready to quit smoking, that person needs an intervention to help; but such an intervention will not be useful for a person who has no desire to quit: That person needs something to show him or her why it would be good to quit. Thus, researchers have used this model as a basis for tailoring interventions to people depending on where they are on a continuum of change.

In your thinking, the conceptualization of your study should come before you develop your proposed intervention or decide what data you will collect. If you are interested in helping people with diabetes manage their disease better, ideally you look at a theory or model and think, "Wow, that theory or model suggests that an intervention should do X or Y, so that is how I need to develop the intervention." For example, the theory of reasoned action (Fishbein & Ajzen, 1975) suggests that people consider the advantages and disadvantages of various options for action and on that basis, make a rational decision about what to do. Such a theory would lead you to recognize that when people do not follow the recommended self-management actions for their diabetes, they have reasons for that, and so you might need to develop an intervention to deal with them. Your conceptual framework would show reasons for not self-managing, an intervention to address those reasons, and expected outcomes.

A major problem is that often other people's models or theories are not actually used by researchers to help them think about what they want to do. Rather, researchers figure out what they want to do and what they think their work will achieve, then look around for a theory or model that will fit the proposed study. That does not help your thinking. You may do it because you need to, but be careful. Sometimes researchers say they are basing their work on theories that are not relevant or helpful, simply because they are available. If you are selecting a theory or model after the fact, at least make sure to select something that will be appropriate for what you are proposing to do.

When you are selecting a theory or model to serve as a guide, it is extremely important to understand that theory or model in detail. It is also important to recognize the difference between using a theory as a framework and drawing on some aspects of the theory in developing your own framework. For example, if you say that a large framework serves as your conceptual framework, but you plan to study only two small variables in the large model, the model is not your conceptual framework. You may have drawn on it to conceptualize your study but you are not using that model. Tell readers what your conceptualization is, and note that you have drawn on the larger model to develop your framework.

If you are planning to test an intervention to reduce risky sex behaviors in young Hispanic girls, doubtless you already know what the risk and protective factors are for these girls. You are not going to identify those; rather, you are going to try to do something new and different to help girls make the best decisions for their lives. So you should not say that your conceptual framework is based on risk and protective factors. You may be drawing on those, but if your new approach builds directly on the strengths of girls' families to help them resist peer pressure, the approach also draws from theory about family dynamics or adolescent development. And it is the new approach itself that is your conceptual framework, not the theories you have drawn from. Your conceptual framework may also guide the design and operationalization of your study. For example, it may suggest what the outcomes should be.

Community-based participatory research (CBPR) is sometimes presented as a framework for a study, but often the intervention planned is not coming from the community but from the researchers who are taking it to the community. They may have a community partner but that is not identical to CBPR. So it is inaccurate to say that CBPR provides your conceptual framework: You may be taking some ideas from it, but you are not doing it.

It is also useful to remember that theories and models come and go. Locus of control (Rotter, 1966) was used in countless studies in the late 20th century, then it disappeared from the scene, though now it seems to be coming back into use. More recently, self-efficacy (Bandura, 1997) has been widely used as a framework for studies, even for studies that did not really seem to be about self-efficacy, and studies in which increasing self-efficacy was not the central goal of the intervention. However, self-efficacy seems to have waned in importance in the past few years. So pay attention to what people are using now.

Begin the description of your conceptual framework with a brief over-view indicating what outcomes you expect and what variables will influ-ence those outcomes. Do you think people will manage their pain better? Lose weight? Take their medicines on time? What variables will influence those outcomes and measure them? If you have an intervention, obviously you expect that to have the major effect on outcomes. So after the over-view, note what effects you think the intervention will have and how they will be measured. Then tell readers whether you expect the intervention to directly affect outcomes, or do so through some intermediary (often called a mediator, but depending on your discipline sometimes termed a modera-tor). For example, do you think the intervention will lower blood glucose levels, or will it improve participants' self-management of diabetes, which will in turn lower glucose levels? You also need to talk about variables that could influence the intervention's effects, usually called moderators. For example, when they enter the study, participants bring with them certain characteristics that may affect the outcomes you expect from an interven-tion, or the relationships you predict among variables. Age, gender, race/ethnicity, education, experience, income, self-efficacy, and other variables all may affect outcomes. Those need to be very briefly described (unless you have already done so in describing the rationale for your study), with ref-erences documenting their importance. However, if you plan to influence any of these variables, they are outcomes, not moderators; they cannot be both. For example, you may plan to improve participants' self-efficacy for caring for children with chronic illnesses. Self-efficacy is thus an outcome variable and you will measure it before and after the intervention to see if it changes. But you cannot also say you will see whether people's self-efficacy before the intervention affects the intervention. That is trying to have it both ways: Intervention affects self-efficacy and self-efficacy affects intervention. The real world may be like that but not research.

Finally, make sure your framework matches your study aims and hypotheses or research questions. For example, if you plan to increase self-efficacy among caregivers who handle wandering Alzheimer's disease patients, that needs to be said not only in the conceptual framework but also in the study aims. Otherwise readers will say the framework is not consistent with the study.

Many reviewers expect you to include a figure illustrating the frame-work (sometimes called a logic model). If you decide to provide a figure, do so after your description of your conceptualization of the study. And the figure must make sense. *Don't be seduced by the infinite possibilities of your design department. Don't go for pretty; go for reasonable.* If you have an intervention, you should not draw a framework in which the arrows go in circles. In an intervention study, the framework is linear. If you have an immensely complicated figure, you may be trying to include too many variables; you need to simplify it enough to make sure both the framework and the study itself make sense. Have a colleague or several colleagues look at the drawing to be sure it makes sense. If you cannot make it make sense, do not include it. Reviewers like to have a drawing, but if it is done wrong, they will hate your proposal.

REFERENCES

Bandura, A. (1997). *Self-efficacy: The exercise of control.* New York, NY: W. H. Freeman.

Fishbein, M., & Ajzen, I. (1975). *Belief, attitude, intention, and behavior: An introduction to theory and research.* Reading, MA: Addison-Wesley.

Huth, E. J. (1999). *Writing and publishing in medicine* (3rd ed.). Philadelphia, PA: Lippincott Williams & Wilkins.

Prochaska, J. O., & DiClemente, C. C. (1982). Transtheoretical therapy: Toward a more integrative model of change. *Psychotherapy: Theory, Research and Practice, 19,* 276–288.

Rotter, J. B. (1966). Generalized expectancies for internal versus external control of reinforcement. *Psychological Monographs: General and Applied, 80*(1), 1–28.

Thomas, L. (1974). *The lives of a cell: Notes of a biology watcher.* New York, NY: The Viking Press.

WORKSHEET FOR DEVELOPING THE RATIONALE FOR YOUR STUDY

To begin, write out your purpose—this is just to get you going: Looking at your purpose will give you the context for developing a rationale for achieving that purpose. Then go through the parts of the argument for a study as listed.

1. THE PROBLEM
   a. Name the overall problem you will be addressing. Is it diabetes? Dementia? Depression? Heart failure? Frailty? Low birth weight?

   b. Document the importance of the problem. Is it serious? Widespread? Growing? Why is it important? Provide at least three references showing importance and briefly summarize the data these articles provide. (You can use the table you created to help you find the best references.) In most proposals, you can make a couple of general statements about importance and then cite all three articles in parentheses; you do not have to describe each one. Now look at what you have said and decide whether you need more data or not.

   c. Next name the aspect of the problem you will be studying. Will you look at unnecessary hospitalizations in patients with heart failure? Or overuse of antipsychotic drugs in nursing home residents with dementia? Do you propose a new intervention to improve self-management of diabetes in a particular group,

(continued)

WORKSHEET FOR DEVELOPING THE RATIONALE FOR
YOUR STUDY (*continued*)

such as Hispanic men? In short, what is the focus of your study? Use your purpose statement to help you specify the particular problem you will work on.

d. Document the importance of this particular aspect of the problem—for example, you might note that a major issue with heart failure is repeated hospitalizations to get rid of severe symptoms such as extreme swelling of the legs and shortness of breath. List references for that statement. Or you might say that in spite of years of efforts to reduce overuse of antipsychotics in dementia patients, a large number of nursing home residents with dementia are still receiving these drugs. Document this.

2. WORK DONE ON THE PROBLEM

   a. Begin with general points about the work done overall. For example, if your area is long-term effects of child abuse, summarize what we know broadly about those effects, with references. If your topic is heart failure, quickly summarize the work that has been done to try to prevent repeated hospitalizations of patients with heart failure.

   b. Indicate how far the work has gone or how successful it has been in general.

   c. Move next to the studies closest to yours, and summarize their findings. For example, if you are planning an innovative approach to engaging children in weight loss, list studies that have used similar approaches and indicate what their effects were. Do not go into details about methods, just point to the findings.

3. SHORTCOMINGS IN THE WORK DONE TO DATE

   a. Point to the reasons why the work to date remains unfinished or needs to be done in a different way. What have the studies closest to yours not done? Did they not look at a population that is growing but about which we know little? Did the interventions they tested show only partial success? Did they have only short-term effects? Why were they only partly successful? Why do you think their effects did not last longer? This is where you list problems with methods— the work has not addressed problem X or population Y, or the interventions did not include X. List all the shortcomings you find. Conclude by providing evidence that the work you plan will do what is needed, succeed where others have failed.

4. PURPOSE

   a. Finally, restate your purpose and see if the points you have made above lead to that purpose and make a compelling case for its potential success. Let others see the case as well, and make it stronger where necessary.

THREE

DESIGN AND METHODS

Whether you are proposing research, an evidence-based practice project, an educational training project, or a demonstration project, you are proposing to do something, and reviewers will expect you to describe the methods that you will use to carry out the work. This is where you talk about your overall approach and make sure readers understand that your approach is appropriate for your project. In this chapter, we provide basic information on what you need to cover in a proposal. However, proposals differ: The National Institutes of Health (NIH) proposals require exquisite detail about research methods; PhD proposals are similar though generally less sophisticated; evidence-based practice projects require some information about methods and, in addition, details about the process you will use to carry out the project; educational research may require detailed information about the faculty and students you will be working with; educational training grant proposals require information about plans for the training and details about the capacity of your institution and the sustainability of your project; and demonstration projects require information about how you will work with the community and continue the project when funding ends. So adapt this basic information to the particular proposal you are planning.

The Methods section should begin with an overview of the research or project, followed by your setting and sample, then the intervention if you have one and your comparison or control group, next a description of how you will collect data on your study variables and, finally, procedures and plans for analysis. It is helpful to keep a notebook on all of the methods decisions that you make as you write this section. Reviewers will not expect a perfect proposal, but they do expect you to have examined alternatives for the methods you decided to use. If you keep notes about alternatives and why you made the choice you made, you will be prepared to explain and that will make your methods stronger.

Specific details about particular types of proposals are provided in the following chapters. We provide the most detail about research methods in the Approach section of Chapter 5 and, therefore, we recommend that you refer to the sections of that chapter to help you plan your study, even if what you are proposing is not as complex as an NIH proposal.

BASIC METHODS

Overview

Sometimes people begin the Methods section by restating the study purpose. Whether you do that should depend on what you have already said. If your purpose is clear, begin the section not with a restatement of purpose but with a brief overview of the design of your study (which is really another way of stating its purpose). This gives readers a framework on which to hang the details of your methods. Some people name the design here and if you are writing a PhD proposal, you may be required to do that. However, remember that giving the design a label is not particularly helpful: People use the same labels to mean different things and different labels to mean the same things. It is more useful to say what you are going to study and why and when. If you are planning an exploratory or descriptive study, say what you will do to collect data on what kinds of people for what purpose. For example, if you are interested in finding out why cardiac patients do not get to the emergency department sooner, you might say, "To identify reasons for delay in seeking treatment for cardiac events, we will ask men and women who delayed seeking treatment what symptoms they experienced, why they delayed seeking treatment, and what made them finally decide to go to the emergency department."

If you are going to test an intervention, say what you will do to determine whether it achieves the outcomes that you are expecting. For example, you might say, "To determine whether an educational intervention on risky sex behaviors reduces these behaviors in adolescent Hispanic girls, we will compare change in the prevalence of these behaviors from baseline to postintervention in a group who receive the intervention and a control group." Perhaps you plan to examine the feasibility and collect beginning evidence of the efficacy of an intervention to reduce obesity in school children. You might introduce your methods with this statement: "We will examine the feasibility of a school-based exercise and diet intervention to reduce obesity in children in grades 4 to 6 by looking at recruitment and retention, ability to carry out the intervention, and participant satisfaction. We will also collect data on the children's weight, body mass index (BMI) and waist circumference at baseline and at follow-up at 6 months after the intervention to determine whether changes occur." That second sentence tells reviewers you know you cannot determine efficacy with one group, but you will get a sense of whether the intervention seems to produce change. If your study is complex, it is often helpful to provide a drawing of your design following the overview; if the study design is simple, however, this is not necessary and wastes space.

Preliminary Work

For some proposals such as PhD proposals and DNP capstone project proposals, you are unlikely to have done preliminary work for your study: This is the beginning. However, for larger studies and studies for which you are requesting funding, you will often have done some preliminary work. If you have done some work to prepare for the proposed study, you need to include it in the proposal. For example, if you plan to test an intervention, you will probably have done some work to decide what the intervention needed to include, perhaps through focus groups with the people targeted for intervention, and you may also have done a pilot of the intervention. That work needs to be described for reviewers—it strengthens the case for your study and shows its potential for success. If you are planning to examine frailty in the elderly, you may have done a review of the literature on this topic and published it. Even if you have not done other work on frailty, this review shows your understanding of the area.

Briefly summarize your prior work, but do not include work you have done in other areas—it is not relevant. And do not describe work done by others: you have described that earlier. Also, if you have done a lot in this area, do not include the work you did initially; reviewers want to know what you did to prepare for the study you are proposing, not what you did long ago in order to begin thinking about it. Briefly summarize each relevant study, as you would for an abstract, though in a little more detail. Do not just say we did some preliminary work and it taught us that we need to do more of X. Reviewers want to know your methods and your findings. It is also useful to have published (or least have "in press") papers on your preliminary work. And if other members of your research team have done work that is important for this study, briefly review that work as well.

Some proposal guidelines may tell you to put preliminary work in a separate section. However, nowadays many people provide a brief summary of their preliminary work after describing the study design or at the very beginning of the Methods section.

We generally recommend that preliminary work follows the Overview of your study, because the Overview helps readers to see the reasons for the preliminary work and its utility. But this is a judgment call: You might try putting the information before and after the overview and see which way seems best. If you are writing a more basic science proposal, you may want to spread the preliminary work throughout the Methods section, since you will have done some preliminary work for the first experiment you plan, and some additional work for the second experiment and so on. In such cases, it is more logical to present the work where it is relevant than to report it all together.

If you have a team who will do the research, you should briefly, very briefly, summarize the expertise of every team member, beginning with you, the principal investigator. (Research assistants are part of the team, but they are not considered investigators so should not be included here.) If this is a big study, you may have several co-investigators; include a sentence or two on the expertise of each. And if you are doing a quantitative study, it is always wise to have a statistician on the team (even if you are good at statistical analysis, unless you have a degree and publications in a statistical area, you need a statistician). We generally recommend that you describe the team first, then go on to describe the preliminary work, because the description of your work leads logically to the study that you are proposing; however, sometimes people choose to put the preliminary work first and then describe the team.

Some proposal guidelines suggest that you list the study hypotheses or research questions after the design overview. If you do so, you might want to put preliminary work before the overview. But you may decide to put hypotheses or questions elsewhere, for example, just after giving your purpose at the end of the section describing the rationale for the study. Use your sense of logic to decide the most appropriate place for these—but never wait until the Analysis section to list them. Readers do not want to suddenly discover what your questions are or find that you have hypotheses at the end of the proposal. We have provided detailed suggestions for writing hypotheses and questions in Chapter 5 and we recommend that you follow them.

Setting(s)

Your settings (or sites) are the places where you will get your subjects and conduct your study. If you plan to conduct an intervention or assess subjects in a setting that is not the same as the one where you will recruit them, first describe the setting where you will recruit subjects, and then talk about where you will conduct the study. Your settings need to be described first, before you describe the sample you expect to recruit. Sometimes people describe their sample first, before saying where they will conduct the study. That puts the cart before the horse. You want first to tell readers enough about your settings to show that you can get the sample you need there. You also want to show that your settings are similar to other, real- world places and thus your work can be used in other places—that is, the study findings will be generalizable. If you are doing educational research, describe the school or department in which you will conduct the study. For *any* clinical setting you plan to use, first say what it is—intensive care unit in a major medical center, a community hospital, federally funded clinic, health department, physician's office, church—and also indicate the type of area it is in—urban, rural, underserved, and so forth—and the kinds of people who are cared for in the setting. A range of people? Mostly minorities? Mostly low-income? Mostly well off? After this brief general description, always indicate that you have a letter from the institution providing you access to participants (and include it in an appendix). Next, indicate how many people the facility serves and how many of these are similar to the patients you need for your study, or how many staff it employs who are similar to the staff members you are seeking as participants. If this is an evidence-based practice project, also give readers some idea about standard procedures in the setting, so readers can tell whether this setting is like others. If you are recruiting minorities for your study, make sure to include figures on the numbers of minorities in the setting.

If you are recruiting subjects in your community, briefly describe the community, including its demographics. And if you are using community agencies for recruitment and perhaps for an intervention, describe those as well; you may also want to make the agency a community partner—be sure in any case to get a letter of support from the agency.

If you plan to intervene or collect data electronically, you will not have a setting but you will need to describe the way you plan to identify potential participants—from a public list, private list, support group, and so forth. Also, think about what your participants will need to do to take part in the study. Perhaps you will expect them to have computers at home, or to use a smartphone (what percentage will have those?). Make clear how you expect participants to access study materials.

Sample

In this section, begin by telling readers the types of persons you will study (children, undergraduate students, the elderly, those with chronic fatigue, etc.) and then list the criteria you will use to select some people and exclude others. First give the inclusion criteria, then the exclusion criteria. Do not, however, simply use the reverse of your inclusion criteria as exclusion criteria: If one inclusion criterion is that participants are older than 65, do not then say you will exclude those younger than 65. That makes you look stupid.

It is easy to figure out whether potential participants meet some criteria, such as age, ethnicity/race and gender, or diagnosis. But you may have to test people to determine whether they meet other criteria; for example, if you want people to be able to follow your instructions and perform certain tasks, you may need to test their cognitive ability using an instrument such as the Mini-Mental State Exam. If participants need to be able to perform certain exercises, you may need to screen them for physical function. If you use an instrument for screening potential participants, describe it here, because it is a screening tool, not a data collection measure. After describing the criteria for including people in the sample, note that you will obtain informed consent from all subjects, and if you are studying children, note that you will get informed consent from parents and assent from the children, if they are old enough to assent.

Next indicate the number of people you intend to enroll and explain the basis for that number. If you have hypotheses, you must have enough participants to test them. We give detailed information about how to determine this in Chapter 5, and we suggest you look at that chapter. For small studies, it is more difficult to decide on the appropriate number. Think about what groups you will have and how many participants you need in each in order to make your findings credible, and then provide the best explanation you can for your decision. (Do not, however, say that you are going to enroll only 20 subjects because this is a dissertation and you will not have time to do more, or you only have money for 20 because this is a small grant. Always provide a scientific explanation for your decision even if it has to do with time or money.) Next, tell readers why you expect to be able to get the number you plan to enroll—perhaps you have done an earlier study that successfully used similar recruitment methods, or others have used this approach successfully.

Then describe your recruitment plans: Who will recruit, when and how. Make sure you include plans for recruiting minorities, who are not always eager to participate in research because of the history of racial discrimination in research or because of fear of immigration authorities or other fears. Also, be sure that your plans for obtaining participants do not conflict with the Health Insurance Portability and Accountability Act (HIPAA) regulations for the protection of patient information. Sometimes people deal with that issue by having clinic or hospital staff describe the proposed study to patients and give the patients a phone number to call if they are interested, but that is not always effective. So think carefully about what you need to do to get subjects and describe your plans fully. And if you are recruiting students for educational research, be careful to avoid pressing them to participate and be sure to protect their confidentiality.

If the study involves more than one data collection point, tell readers what you will do to keep people in the study. Your efforts may include ways to keep in touch with people such as holiday cards and birthday cards or a newsletter about the study, and ways to contact people if they don't show up for an intervention session or for data collection. You may also include an incentive for participation; if so, be sure it is adequate but not so large as to be coercive. Also indicate what kind of attrition you expect in spite of these efforts. You want to keep attrition to no more than 20% because if it gets much above that, you are not likely to get credible findings. You also need to show why you expect attrition to be in that range—perhaps you were able to retain the sample in some earlier work you did, or work by others shows that your methods are likely to succeed.

If you are doing a qualitative study, use an approach for describing the setting and sample that is similar to that for a quantitative study: Describe the setting in which you will recruit participants, the types of participants you will recruit, the method you will use to recruit them, and the sample size you estimate. Also note that this sample size might be adjusted during the course of the study.

Next, if you have groups—for example, an intervention and a control or comparison group—tell readers how you will assign people to those groups. It is important to show readers that you are not putting all the weak students in the control group and the strong students in the intervention group, or the very sick patients in the control group and the not-so-sick ones in the intervention group—or no one will believe you when you say those in the intervention group were better at follow-up than the control group. Therefore, you will probably use some kind of randomization method for putting people in groups. But remember that randomization does not always guarantee that groups are similar, so you may have to look at differences in the groups when you analyze your data.

Intervention

If your study is not an intervention study, go straight from the sample description to Data Collection. However, note that all evidence-based practice projects include an intervention: You are intervening to help providers use evidence in their practice. (While demonstration projects are not considered research, a demonstration is really an intervention, so think about following the basic methods for interventions in describing your project.) If you are studying an intervention, it is helpful to begin with a brief overview of what you will do, to provide the reader with a skeleton on which to hang the details that follow. This is especially important if the intervention is complex, because readers can easily get lost in the details. And always describe what you will do for the intervention group before describing what you will do for the control or comparison group.

After giving the overview of the intervention, describe the bases for what you plan to do. Your intervention may be based on the conceptual framework you presented in the introductory rationale for your study, or you may have already developed and tested the intervention for feasibility and beginning efficacy and you are now planning a more definitive test of efficacy. Or the intervention you plan to look at may be based on the literature; that is, someone else may have developed and tested the intervention, and you are adapting it to a different population or situation. Or maybe your intervention is based on a qualitative study in which you asked patients what they needed in the way of information, support, and so forth.

Next describe the intervention. You will have one small challenge here. If you have done preliminary work to develop or test the intervention, you need to describe that work somewhere, probably in the section on Preliminary Work at the beginning of Methods. Your challenge is deciding whether to describe the intervention fully in Preliminary Work, or save the description for the Methods section. There are advantages and disadvantages either way. If you describe the intervention in Preliminary Work and show that it was feasible and you found beginning evidence of efficacy, it will strengthen the argument for the more definitive study of the intervention you are proposing. But then you will repeat yourself if you describe it in the Intervention section. If you do not describe the intervention in Preliminary Work, your background is weaker, but you can present the intervention here in detail. You have to decide which is the better approach and try to maximize its advantages.

Next tell readers what you propose to do for your intervention or experimental group. Begin with an overview or summary of the content that will be covered. And tell readers how you will organize that content— sequentially, or with multiple topics in a session, with half of each session for education and half for practice, or some other organization.

Then provide details on the content of the intervention. For example, if you plan to conduct family sessions on hypertension risks among African Americans and ways to reduce risks, tell readers what those sessions will include—perhaps information about smoking, diet, lack of exercise, stress, and so forth, and then information about how to take small steps to improve diet and increase activity, ways to support each other in engaging in change, and ways to sustain change. You might also plan some exercise sessions and provide instructions on carrying out exercises at home; describe those as well. If this is an evidence-based practice project, you may plan to engage staff in the neonatal intensive care unit in helping mothers of low-birth-weight infants breastfeed. Say how you are going to show these nurses and doctors the evidence that this is important, and how you are going to engage them in doing what is needed by mothers. Perhaps you plan to provide staff with research materials, hold educational sessions for them, and provide criteria for deciding which infants should be breastfed, and then demonstrate the process and monitor outcomes. Give readers the details they need.

Also, if you will offer boosters or follow-ups of some sort, say whether they will be a part of the intervention, or if they will be given only to a subgroup, and you will compare outcomes of this group to a group that does not get boosters. Finally, if your intervention group will receive usual care, as with the comparison or control group, note that.

Sometimes you will want to tailor an intervention to individuals or to specific groups. For example, if you give participants a pretest on their knowledge of self-care for diabetes and this shows that some persons know how to monitor their glucose level but not how to do foot care, you may wish to focus on foot care with such persons. Others might need information on glucose monitoring and still others might need information in both areas. While tailoring recognizes that individuals differ in their needs, the challenge of tailoring is that not everyone is going to get the same intervention, so you have to figure out how you will evaluate outcomes and make that clear to readers.

The intervention needs to be described in enough detail to enable readers to decide whether it is likely to be efficacious. Readers also want to know whether the intervention is feasible for staff and for patients, and whether it will be so long or complex as to be burdensome. Finally, readers want to know whether the intervention will be usable in other settings. Even if the intervention works, if it can only be done in special settings, it may not be worth funding. So if you are seeking funding for your study, it is essential to provide these details. If you are not sure whether you have provided enough details, ask a colleague to look at your description and give you some feedback. Then you will know whether you have enough or need more.

You also need to tell readers how you will deliver the intervention—in person, electronically, by phone, by some other means. It is particularly important to make this clear in translational research projects, and more specifically, evidence-based practice projects. If the intervention is delivered in person, will it be offered to individuals or groups? If in groups, where will they meet? When? Who will make sure the participants can get there? If delivered individually, will you go to the participant's home or meet elsewhere? And if you are working with professionals, will you intervene with them on the unit or in the agency or somewhere else? Think through all these aspects of the proposed intervention and describe them in your proposal.

It is also important to tell readers who will deliver the intervention. If you are testing an innovative educational strategy, you must indicate whether the faculty who will use this strategy are the same faculty who will be using the traditional method, or different people. If they are the same, how will you prevent contamination? If they are different, are they comparable?

For clinical interventions, it is important to show that the skills and background of interveners are appropriate for the intervention. If there is going to be only one intervener, you have to worry about whether effects are due to the intervention or the intervener. If you have more than one intervener, it is important to ensure that all of the people delivering the intervention do so in exactly the same way. That is why people have a protocol for interveners to follow. It is also helpful to provide training to the interveners and have them practice delivering the intervention to people similar to those who will receive the intervention. Then you will need to monitor their delivery of the intervention and retrain people who do not meet certain criteria for effectiveness.

If you have a very complex intervention, you may need interveners to be highly educated. But if you require these highly educated individuals to deliver your intervention and they are unlikely to be available in the real world, your intervention may never be used. Thus, people often first test an intervention using interveners with an advanced educational background, then, if the intervention is efficacious under these ideal conditions, they try to see whether it works when delivered by the care providers who are available for a particular population—public health department staff or social workers or even lay health workers. (The first proposal is to test efficacy, and the next proposal is to test effectiveness.)

Control or Comparison Group

If you have an intervention, a major question is what you are going to do for the control or comparison group: Will they receive usual care? And what is the usual care in your setting? You may want to provide some sort of "attention" to the control group to match the attention to the intervention group. However, this can be challenging because attention is sometimes a part of an intervention, even though not acknowledged as such, or you could give the control group such an interesting alternative to the intervention that they improve without your intervention. To avoid these issues, you may plan to compare your intervention group to a group of individuals who were in the same setting before the intervention. But you do not know whether their situation was similar to that of your group and this may affect your outcomes. Clearly, there are advantages and disadvantages to any type of comparison or control condition; try to find the best one, although none may be ideal.

Variables and Their Measurement

This section of your proposal describes the measures you will use to answer your questions about the problem you are studying or test the efficacy of your intervention. As with the intervention, it is helpful to begin with a very brief list of the variables you will be assessing. Then, to save space, you can provide a table that lists the variables you will measure and briefly summarize the measures you will use. Make sure to include measures for every variable you will study. Any instruments you use should have established reliability and validity, and be appropriate for your particular population. Also, you need to tell readers how long it takes to administer/complete each instrument. If you have developed an instrument yourself, you will need to report some preliminary work on appropriateness and psychometrics before submitting a proposal that uses the instrument.

You might also use physiological measures, take biological samples, use observational approaches, or administer open-ended questions or structured interviews, conduct document reviews, and so forth. If you are going to use physiological measures, you need to say what they are, what exactly they measure, what evidence there is that they reliably measure what you want to measure, how you will carry out the measurements, and who will do that. If you plan to collect biological samples, you need to say what samples you will collect, who will collect them and how, and where and how they will be analyzed. (Do not save that information for the Human Subjects section: It is a part of your Methods. In Human Subjects, you will talk about how you plan to protect participants from any harm that might occur in the sample collection.) If you plan to observe people's behavior, tell readers what you will observe, who will make the observations, how you will record the observations, how you will score or analyze them and who will do that analysis. If you are looking at something that is not precisely defined, say how you will interpret what you see. If you plan to use open-ended questions, tell readers what they are—or at least list the topics to be covered. And if you plan structured or semi-structured interviews, say what questions you plan to ask or what types of information you are trying to gain. If you plan to review documents such as medical records, indicate what you will be looking for, who will do the review, and how you will deal with missing or unclear data. Each approach needs to be presented in the same order. Finally, if you are not collecting all the data yourself, you need to say how you will train data collectors and ensure that they collect the data you need, do it in the same way, and avoid missing data.

If you are planning a qualitative study, you need to give some indication of what approach you will take. First, think about what you are trying to find out from this study. Then describe how you will get the data you are looking for. For example, if you want to find out what information or support older women with diabetes need in order to better manage their disease, you probably want to ask them some specific questions about their problems and needs and to propose a content analysis, not a phenomenological study. If you plan a phenomenological study, note that all experience is lived experience so you don't have to say "lived," and you need to indicate what this study is likely to tell you that will be important for health. Describing people's experience is not enough. Qualitative work is fundable, but it is exploratory work, and therefore it is important to say what you expect it to lead to: either development of an instrument to broadly test people such as those you have interviewed, or development of an intervention to deal with the issues you have discovered.

Procedures

This section explains how you will take each person through the study, from recruitment through data collection. However, this section overlaps with other aspects of your methods in many ways, and if you are short of space, you can omit Procedures. Just make sure you have covered all of the relevant material elsewhere. For example, Procedures usually includes information on how you will recruit participants and obtain informed consent for those who are eligible and willing to participate. If you have already described your recruitment plans and said that you would gain informed consent in the Sample section, you do not need to repeat the information here. Similarly, if you have indicated how and where you will provide the intervention, how and when you will collect data, and what you will do to ensure that participants remain in the study, do not say all that again. One way to decide whether you need this section is to first write it, then check it against the information you have already provided. If you see a lot of repetition, you can move a little more information to the Sample section and other relevant sections and omit Procedures. However, if there is a lot of new information in Procedures, keep the section and move anything that is really procedural from earlier sections to this section. Some proposal guidelines may require Procedures; if so, try to make sure that you are not just repeating yourself.

Plans for Data Management and Analysis

The Analysis section may be the hardest part of a proposal to write unless you are a whiz at statistics. It is helpful to get some consultation from a statistician, and if you are writing a proposal for funding, ask a statistician to join the research team. Then that person can write this section. We give detailed suggestions for analysis plans in Chapter 5 and we recommend that you look at that chapter before writing this section.

In brief, begin by telling reviewers how you will ensure that the data you analyze are accurate and reasonably complete. And if you expect some missing data, tell readers how you will handle that issue.

Then say what you will do to describe your sample. If you have an intervention and control or comparison group, say what variables you will use to compare them. Then tell readers what you will do if there are differences. In describing your measures, if you have stated that you will conduct reliability and validity checks on some of the instruments you use, make sure to say here what you will do to check those psychometrics.

Then indicate how you will test hypotheses and/or answer research questions. If you have both hypotheses and questions, describe plans for testing hypotheses first. Always repeat or summarize each hypothesis or question. You may know them so well you could recite them in your sleep, but no one else remembers them and readers hate having to look back to some earlier section to figure out what you are analyzing. Go through the analysis one hypothesis or question at a time. For each, first tell readers what variables you will use and then what statistical approach you will take. Select the most appropriate approach, which may not be the fanciest. When you describe your approach, do not give readers a lesson in statistics. You do not need to inform them about how this approach works unless it is very new or would not be thought appropriate for your data without some explanation. If you are taking the same approach for each hypothesis, do not repeat the description of the approach each time; simply tell readers that you will use the same approach as for earlier hypotheses, with differences based on the different variables you will be using.

If your study is qualitative, describe what you will do to analyze the data, but do not give a textbook explanation of the method you will be using. Tell readers what you will do with your particular data. And make sure to describe your plans for ensuring the credibility of your findings.

WRAP UP

Finally, review all the parts of your Methods section and make sure that they are consistent with each other and with your overall purpose. Sometimes people make a change in one part of the proposal but forget to note it elsewhere. You do not want to say that you will collect data on 30 people in your Sample section and then say you will assign people to one of the two groups, with 10 people in the intervention group and 10 in the control group. Check your data collection methods against what you say you hope to achieve with the intervention. Make sure that the data you are collecting cover all the variables mentioned in your hypotheses or research questions and that you have plans for analyzing all the data. Check everything again and again. The more you review and edit your work, the better it becomes.

WORKSHEET FOR DEVELOPING THE DESIGN AND METHODS FOR YOUR STUDY

PURPOSE

In order to (specify the purpose)

_____

_____

_____

_____

_____

DESIGN

Comparison versus relationship versus descriptive (or more than one of these)

COMPARE GROUPS	RELATE VARIABLES	DESCRIBE
What groups?	What variables?	What variables?
Randomly assigned to groups?	In whom?	In whom?
What to compare them on?	At what points in time?	At what points in time?
At what points in time?	Compare relationships?	Examining patterns?

Graphic depiction of your design (does not necessarily need to be included in what you write), but do draw it out here.

Where will you recruit subjects? (Or, where were they recruited, if secondary data.)

For each recruitment setting (site) describe:

Where the site is located:
Type of facility:
Who they serve (Health variables relevant to your study: e.g., geographical, racial/ethnic, gender, age):

(continued)

WORKSHEET FOR DEVELOPING THE DESIGN AND METHODS FOR YOUR STUDY (*continued*)

How many they serve similar to your subjects:

Access (Have you been granted access? Refer to support letter in appendix.):

For each conduct setting (site) (e.g., intervention, data collection) describe:

Relevant characteristics:

Access (Have you been granted access? Refer to support letter in appendix.):

SAMPLE

Whom you will be studying:

Inclusion/exclusion criteria:

How the subjects will be selected:

(continued)

**WORKSHEET FOR DEVELOPING THE DESIGN AND METHODS
FOR YOUR STUDY (*continued*)**

Number you plan to recruit:

Basis for number you plan to recruit:

Attrition estimates (if studying over time):

Flow of subjects through the study:
  To help you figure out the number you plan to recruit, calculate the following:
  • Number available per setting (site): _____
  • Percent of those available you anticipate will meet your criteria: _____
  • Percent of those who meet criteria you will approach/recruit: _____
  • Percent of those you approach anticipated to agree: _____
  • Percent of those who agree anticipated to qualify once screened: _____
  • Resulting number: _____
  • Percent anticipated attrition (if study is more than one time point): _____
  • Number anticipated to complete the study: _____
  Note—there has to be a basis for these numbers—you can't just make them up.

How will subjects be assigned to groups (if relevant)?

Recruitment plans:

Minority recruitment plans:

(continued)

**WORKSHEET FOR DEVELOPING THE DESIGN AND METHODS
FOR YOUR STUDY (*continued*)**

Retention plans:

If you are doing a qualitative study:

Sampling principle you are using:

Inclusion/exclusion criteria:

Estimated number you think you might have:

Basis for this number:

How you will determine when you have a sufficient number:

INTERVENTION

Theory, conceptualization, principles:

(*continued*)

**WORKSHEET FOR DEVELOPING THE DESIGN AND METHODS
FOR YOUR STUDY (*continued*)**

Content:
Structure:
Magnitude:
Delivery issues:
Documenting delivery:
Maintaining integrity:
Control/comparison Group(s)?

Design/content of intervention: If complex, add figure or table(s):

VARIABLES AND MEASURES
- What will you measure/assess?
- How you will measure/assess it?

(*continued*)

**WORKSHEET FOR DEVELOPING THE DESIGN AND METHODS
FOR YOUR STUDY (*continued*)**

- When you will measure/assess it?
- Characteristics of:
  - Formal measures (instruments)?
  - Physiological measures?
  - Biological measures?
  - Observations?
  - Open-ended questions?
  - Structured interviews?
  - Document review?
- Make a table of your data collection approaches (adapt the following to suit your study; include more columns if you can get additional information in the table):

VARIABLES	MEASURES/ INSTRUMENTS (AND CITATION)	PSYCHOMETRICS/ MEASUREMENT CHARACTERISTICS	ADMINISTRATION TIME POINTS
Outcomes:			
Predictors:			
Mediators/ moderators:			
Subject characteristics:			
Other:			

PROCEDURES

If not included in other sections, tell a story—describe the process for each subject. For example:

Identification of subjects:

Initial contact:

(*continued*)

**WORKSHEET FOR DEVELOPING THE DESIGN AND METHODS
FOR YOUR STUDY (*continued*)**

Baseline data collection:

Assignment to groups:

Intervention contacts:

Additional data collection contacts:

Time commitments (subject burden):

Incentives:

Retention contacts/activities:

(continued)

**WORKSHEET FOR DEVELOPING THE DESIGN AND METHODS
FOR YOUR STUDY (*continued*)**

PLANS FOR DATA ANALYSIS

Data management?

Preliminary analyses?

Test/evaluate first hypothesis/research question:

Restate/paraphrase:

Specify variables and statistical test(s) or analysis approach:

Test/evaluate second hypothesis/research question:

Restate/paraphrase:

Specify variables and statistical test(s) or analysis approach:

(continued)

**WORKSHEET FOR DEVELOPING THE DESIGN AND METHODS
FOR YOUR STUDY (*continued*)**

Test/evaluate third hypothesis/research question:

Restate/paraphrase:
Specify variables and statistical test(s) or analysis approach:

For more "qualitative" aspects discuss:

Data management quality:
Information extraction/data coding:
Analytic process and documentation:
Exploring relationships:
Verification of interpretation:

SECTION II: TYPES OF PROPOSALS

FOUR

PhD PROPOSALS

THE TRADITIONAL APPROACH

The essential reasons for writing a PhD dissertation proposal are: first, you want to learn how to write a research proposal, so that you can later write winning proposals for funding or, if not funding, approval; second, you want to propose research that you will conduct in coming months that is useful in itself and also provides a basis for later, larger studies. Many schools and departments of nursing and other health professions use a three-chapter traditional format for writing a PhD proposal: Chapter I presents the rationale for the study, Chapter II is a review of the literature, and Chapter III describes the proposed study methods. However, there are some problems with this approach. If you have to follow it, it is useful to understand these problems.

First, the traditional dissertation proposal is often quite long, with Chapter II running 50 or more pages. Yet the proposals you write for funding are much shorter. As we have noted in the chapter on National Institutes of Health (NIH) proposals, R03 and R21 proposals are usually seven single-spaced pages (one page for Specific Aims and six pages for Research Strategy), and R15 and R01 proposals are 13 pages (one page for Specific Aims and 12 pages for Research Strategy). Proposals for foundations are also short. Thus, to succeed in gaining funding, it is important to learn to write succinct proposals. Writing a lengthy dissertation proposal doesn't help you develop the skill. Further, the lengthy dissertation proposal (and dissertation) is one reason why doctoral study in nursing tends to be longer than in many other disciplines. There is increasing interest in making doctoral study in nursing move faster, and writing a shorter proposal would help in that regard, both for students and faculty members who advise them and must read all those pages.

Further, the traditional format often contains a great deal of overlap between the first two chapters and does not give you practice in making a coherent argument for a study. In any dissertation proposal, as in other proposals, the argument for the study is the standard argument described earlier in this book: There is a problem, some work has been done on the problem, but the work has not gone far enough or been done right, and therefore this study takes the work further or does it right. Logically, this rationale is based on the literature: Building on what has already been done, the study extends the work to a new population or problem, or it delves deeper into a problem we already know about, or uses more rigorous methods or more appropriate interventions to solve the problem. Thus, literature forms the basis for the argument. You want to make this argument in your first chapter of the proposal, but the traditional format puts the literature in a different chapter, so that you either have to say the same things twice or try to make the case for your study without referring to the literature that is the basis for the study. That is one reason why Chapter I is so hard to write.

Also, the traditional Chapter I often contains sections that are unnecessary or confusing and these make the chapter choppy. For example, frequently there is a section called Problem Statement in addition to the Purpose, but this problem statement is really a different way of stating the study purpose, not a description of the problem. The first chapter may also include a section called Significance, but that is redundant: The significance of the proposed work should already be clear from your description of why the study is needed. Chapter I may also include a section called Assumptions and one on Limitations. But your assumptions should be clear in your description of the conceptualization of your work, and the limitations of your proposed methods should be mentioned where they are relevant. For example, if there are limitations to the sampling methods you use, they need to be discussed with the information on sampling in the chapter on methods. Here they are meaningless because there is no context for them.

Many of these proposals also include sections on definitions and a list of abbreviations. Any word that needs to be defined should be defined in text the first time it is used. That is when readers want to know its meaning, not 10 pages later in a separate section. For example, if you are going to study cancer survivors, say right away what you mean by survivor. Is a survivor anyone who has had a cancer diagnosis and is still alive? Is a survivor a person who has finished treatment? Or lived for a certain number of years posttreatment? Readers want to know this before going further.

Readers also want to know the terms you are using right away; if you are going to use an abbreviation, always spell out the word the first time it appears, with the abbreviation following in parentheses. Readers don't want to have to look it up on a list to find out whether you are talking about advance directive or Alzheimer's disease when you use AD. (In the PhD proposal, or any other proposal, don't abbreviate the names of groups of people: It is dehumanizing to use AA for African Americans or KA instead of Korean Americans. If you need to save space, you should do it another way.)

Finally, the traditional organization makes it hard to write articles reporting the dissertation research. Graduates find it enormously difficult to cut and focus the literature review in Chapter II. As a result, many do not publish their dissertation work—a great waste—and those who do publish often follow an outdated organization based on the dissertation format. That is, their articles often begin with an Introduction making the case for the study and giving its purpose, followed by a section called Background or Review of the Literature that doesn't seem to have much to do with anything, and then perhaps a description of the theoretical framework, which may or may not be relevant, and finally the purpose again. That comes from the organization of the proposal and dissertation: Chapter I, Argument, Chapter II, Literature Review, and Chapter III, Methods. Most biomedical journals now include only a short introduction in research articles that briefly makes the case for study, and many other health care journals are moving in that direction as well. This Introduction is almost like the specific aims page for an NIH proposal; it is not like the dissertation proposal. Thus the organization of a dissertation proposal teaches you to write in a way that not only makes it hard to get funded for your research, but also makes it hard to get published after you have done the research. There is something wrong with this picture.

You may need to follow the traditional format, but it is useful to your thinking to understand its illogicalities, even if you have to conform to them. One way to understand these is to recognize that some of the traditional requirements are really not requirements for a standard proposal, but exercises to make sure you show that you know what you are doing. In other words, your proposal is not designed to inform readers (your dissertation committee), but to inform readers that you are informed. For example, Chapter II is designed to show your committee that you have conducted a comprehensive review of the literature in your area. If you must include a section on definitions, that section is designed to show that you know the meanings of the terms that you are using, and if you have to include a section titled Significance, that is designed to make sure you understand why this study is important. The more you think about the rationale for your study, the more you will be able to provide sophisticated rather than simplistic information for your committee, whether you use the traditional format or a different approach. We suggest three different approaches to help you write a more coherent, concise dissertation proposal, which you might try. If that is not possible, think, think, and think again about what you are doing in the traditional proposal and why, and write it in the most concise, clear way you can.

THREE DIFFERENT APPROACHES

The National Research Service Award Proposal

The first suggestion is to ask your advisor or dissertation chair to allow you to write your dissertation proposal in the form of a National Research Service Award (NRSA) fellowship proposal to the NIH. The NRSA proposal is for both research and training so you must include a training plan in addition to proposing a study, but the NRSA is well suited to doctoral study and dissertation work. We give specific suggestions for writing any NIH proposal in Chapter 5 and for writing an NRSA proposal in Chapter 6. Writing this proposal helps you build the skills you need to gain funding later, and if you submit the proposal and are funded, the fellowship supports your dissertation study. The NRSA proposal also looks extremely good on your résumé, and if you don't get funded, you will get very helpful critiques from reviewers, which will enable you to strengthen your work. Finally, writing this kind of proposal may not make your writing time any shorter (writing a proposal for funding can take several drafts), but it will cut your dissertation committee's reading time and help prepare you for a career as a researcher.

The Traditional Proposal in Two Chapters

The second suggestion is this: If you decide to write a traditional dissertation proposal, ask your advisor to let you try doing it in only two chapters; that is, develop the rationale for your study in Chapter I and describe your proposed study methods in Chapter II. You might title Chapter I "Background and Purpose" or "The Rationale for the Study." Follow the suggestions for developing the rationale for your study that we provided in Chapter 2. Start with a description of the problem you are addressing, and cite the literature to provide evidence of its importance. It may be helpful to put this description under a subheading such as "The Prevalence of Asthma in Children," or "Heart Failure in the Elderly." Begin with the big problem—asthma or depression or diabetes or delirium or whatever the overall issue is. Remember, however, that the better known the problem, the less literature you need to cite to convince readers of its importance.

After you have presented the overall problem, move on to the specific aspect of the problem you will be studying. You may need another subheading here: "Asthma in Low-Income Children," "Pain in Nursing Home Residents With Dementia," "Depression in Adolescent Victims of Dating Violence," or "Self-Management of Diabetes by American Indians," or

"Delirium in the Elderly Following Orthopedic Surgery." Here again, use the literature to document the specific problem you will address.

Next, describe what has been done about the problem. We provided suggestions for synthesizing the literature in Chapter 2, and these will be helpful to you in organizing this section of the proposal. You might use a subheading here, "Studies of Diabetes in American Indians" or whatever the problem is for your population, or "Interventions for Reducing Risky Sex Behaviors in Hispanic Early Adolescents." This is where you give more details about the literature in order to show what you are building on and why more work is needed. First, describe the general literature in a few sentences, with references (e.g., in a sentence such as this: "Numerous studies have documented the high prevalence of diabetes in Hispanics [reference, reference, reference]"), then move on to studies that are directly related to what you are planning. You don't need to go into detail about studies that are not directly related to your work and you don't need to summarize every study. For example, if you are planning to try a new approach to providing HIV testing and counseling to prostitutes working around army bases, talk briefly about general approaches to reach the hard-to-reach for HIV testing with several references, then focus on studies reporting efforts that have been made to provide testing and counseling for the specific group you are interested in. Then discuss the extent of success of those efforts and, finally, point out why a new study is needed. Perhaps no one has focused on this particular group and you will need to extrapolate information from other groups, or perhaps the methods tried with this group were not appropriate. You might want to review the suggestions in Chapter 2 for making these points, and remember, you want to credit the achievements of the work that has already been done but also make clear its shortcomings.

Most dissertation committees want to make sure that students have done a comprehensive review of the literature, but the rationale for a study is not designed to be a comprehensive summary of the literature. If your committee members wish to see evidence of your full grasp of the literature in your area, you can construct a table showing everything you have read, giving author, title, publication date, purpose, methods, findings, and conclusions for each study. You can attach that as an appendix to the dissertation proposal or you can write a state of the science paper that reviews the literature in your area. We make suggestions for this in the section on the "Three-Chapter Approach" that follows. If no one has published such a review in the last few years, you will certainly be able to publish it. Remember that if we want evidence-based practice, the best way to get the evidence to practitioners is to publish review papers.

Your analysis of the literature should lead logically to the purpose of the study you are proposing. We recommend that you use a subheading here: "Purpose, Aims, and Hypotheses" (or "Research Questions"). State the purpose, and if you have specific aims or objectives, state those under the purpose. Then state your hypotheses and/or research questions. However, check the suggestions in Chapter 5 on NIH research grant proposals so that you don't mistakenly propose hypotheses when you won't have a sample big enough to test them.

Also, don't state aims and questions or hypotheses that are identical For example, our first aim is to determine whether individuals with HIV infection are more likely than others to suffer fatigue; our hypothesis is that those with HIV infection are significantly more likely than other individuals to suffer fatigue; and our research question is, do individuals with HIV suffer more fatigue than other individuals?

After you have given your purpose, specific aims, and hypotheses and/or questions, describe the conceptual framework for the study if you have a conceptual framework. We made some suggestions for presenting a conceptual framework in Chapter 2. This discussion should end the chapter.

You are ready now for Chapter II, "Study Methods." This chapter will be similar whether you use the traditional format or the two-chapter format or the different three-chapter format we are suggesting. We made detailed suggestions for presenting your study methods in Chapter 3. Follow those suggestions and use the worksheet included at the end of the chapter to develop Chapter II. Be as rigorous as you can, but remember that this is a dissertation proposal, not a major study, and you want to finish it in a reasonable amount of time. Think of this as an exploratory or feasibility or pilot study, with limits on what you can expect to achieve. For example, you may have learned a lot about power analysis in your research courses, but if you need to collect data from 150 families in order to test hypotheses and that is unreasonable in the timeframe you have, don't test hypotheses. Work with your advisor or dissertation chair to develop reasonable methods, and seek help from other experts in your area. Be clear about what you will do and show that the study will provide a foundation for more definitive work. Above all, don't promise more than you can deliver in a reasonable time, or you will be doing this forever—or you won't finish.

A Different Three-Chapter Approach

If your program or advisor requires the three-chapter approach, first write Chapter I as we have suggested previously, making the case for your study and leaving out unnecessary little sections. (Remember that your advisor wants you to be aware of the need to define your terms, understand your assumptions, recognize what the problem is, etc., but you can show this knowledge without having to put it in little boxes.)

In the traditional dissertation format, Chapter II is the review of the literature. However, if you have made a compelling argument for your study in Chapter I, you have already used the literature. So you need to do something different in Chapter II. Instead of writing a lengthy comprehensive literature review for Chapter II, try writing a review paper synthesizing the work you have examined and drawing conclusions about the state of the science and the work that remains to be done. You can still call it Chapter II. This may give you a publication that shows your grasp of the literature in the area both to your committee as well as to general readers, and that publication will be useful when you seek funding for further research.

This review paper should report current research in your area; it is designed to show the state of the science. To write a review paper, you must read a great deal, but when you write the paper, don't summarize everything you have read. Most review papers are no longer than 15 to 18 pages. (As we noted previously, if you feel you must show your committee that you have a grasp of all the literature, you can do a summary table of all the studies you examined and attach this as an appendix to the dissertation—but don't include that in the paper to be submitted for publication; in that paper you may include a table, but only of the work that you have included in the review.)

If you write Chapter II as a review paper, you need to be clear that this paper is different from a review of the literature designed to develop the rationale for your study. When you use the literature to develop the rationale for a study, you are focusing on the need for that particular study. But a review paper is not about the rationale for a particular study: It is about what we know about a problem or its solutions. There are basically two types of review articles: When a good deal of work has been done on solutions, the review is designed to tell readers what can be concluded from research and put into practice now. This type of paper may also note areas about which we do not know enough to draw conclusions and may suggest more research in those areas. Review papers like these are extremely helpful in getting research into practice. Thus, they are frequently published in practice journals, such as nurse practitioner journals, though they may not be called review articles.

When research is more exploratory, a review paper is designed to show what research has been done on the problem, what it has accomplished, and what questions still need to be addressed. The review is not designed to lead to practice but to further research. Thus, research journals may be more interested in this type of review article. These articles are also more difficult to write because you have to be very clear about the research to date—and that may mean looking at literature from multiple disciplines. You cannot assume that because nothing has been done in your discipline, nothing has been done.

Before beginning your article, think about what type of review article it is and what your conclusions are from reading the literature. Then, in your article, organize the literature in a way that leads readers to draw the conclusions you have reached based on the findings of the studies you reviewed and the adequacy of their methods, and thus the credibility of the findings.

Always begin the review paper (Chapter II) by presenting the problem. However, don't go on and on about the problem; quickly summarize general descriptions and then focus on the aspect of the problem you are interested in. For example, if the review paper is about the influence of low health literacy on the failure of African Americans to follow treatment regimens for heart disease, first briefly describe the high burden of heart disease among African Americans and then point to studies showing that one reason for their poor outcomes is failure to follow treatment regimens. Note that, in order to effectively intervene, we must understand why African Americans do not follow treatment regimens, and conclude the discussion by saying that one possible reason is low health literacy in this group. Provide references for all these statements, and say that this paper discusses studies that have examined the effects of low health literacy on African Americans' failure to follow these regimens, or whatever your focus is.

Then describe the search methods and criteria you used for including studies in the review. Begin by indicating what databases you used and what search terms. Then list the criteria for inclusion; for example, you reviewed studies that included African Americans with advanced heart disease, looked at level of adherence to medications, and looked at health literacy. You included only studies published in the last decade, in English. You did not include opinion pieces or anecdotal data. Make your reasons for these criteria clear. Why only advanced disease? Why only studies in the previous decade? What about studies that included both African Americans and Caucasians? Why no anecdotal data? Did the studies have to give a definition of health literacy?

Indicate how many studies you retrieved and how many met the criteria for review. Then give an overview of the findings of the studies, starting with the most general and moving toward those more specific to the area of interest, the influence of health literacy on adherence or whatever your specific topic is. It is important to summarize the most important findings of the studies; don't just say they had findings, but don't summarize everything the authors say either. You want to report what matters, both from the authors' perspectives and from yours. The concluding discussion of a study report should indicate what the authors think is important, though as noted in Chapter 2, authors sometimes fail to indicate their conclusions, concentrating instead on their limitations. One way to check their view of importance is to look at what findings the authors note in the abstract, though that too can be vague. Thus, you need to think about what is important. Also, if studies have had conflicting findings, point this out; if they overlap, point this out. Include a table or matrix showing the details of the studies (authors, journal, publication date, sample, methods, including the intervention if they were intervention studies, findings, and conclusions).

Next, give an overall evaluation of the quality of the evidence provided by these studies (don't describe the methods study by study; that will be in the table). Do this evaluation carefully, not by checklist. For example, if some of the studies did not have a theoretical framework, you cannot simply say that these studies were therefore inadequate; rather, you need to look at the conceptualization of the studies and decide whether a theoretical framework was needed. Note that the more physiological a study is, the less likely it is to have a labeled theoretical framework. You cannot simply say that some studies had a small sample, and therefore were not adequate. Suppose the studies were examining ventilator-associated pneumonia in patients in intensive care. What kind of sample is possible for these patients? The key is to use your common sense in deciding what flaws are important in studies and what flaws are not fatal. Finally, say what we can conclude for practice, if this is the first type of review, and point out what remains to be done. If it is the second type of review, point out what we now definitively know and what remains unclear and needs more study.

In writing a review paper, especially if this is your first, it is helpful to make an outline of your points to be sure that your review is logical and coherent. It is also helpful to find a published review article that you like and use it as a template. Carefully examine the authors' organization and emphases and use those to guide your own organization. But make sure the article you follow is one that makes sense to you; don't try to follow an organization that you think is incoherent. Because you will be thinking about publication, after the first draft cut out peripheral work and condense to 15 to 18 pages.

DEVELOPING THE PROPOSAL

Whether you use the two- or three-chapter approach to a dissertation proposal, these suggestions should guide you. If you do an NRSA proposal for the dissertation, follow the same guidelines but make your rationale more concise, following NIH guidelines.

As noted, your chapter on methods will be more or less the same whether you use the two- or three-chapter approach. Much of your work in developing the proposal will be working on methods. Developing the argument for the study is a relatively solitary task, but you will want to confer frequently with your advisor or chair about the methods. We made detailed suggestions for methods development in Chapter 3, and there is a worksheet at the end of the chapter to help you specify your methods. Also, Chapter 5 on NIH research grant proposals contains additional details about methods. However, it is important to remember that this is a pilot study or an exploratory study; it is not the definitive work in your area. You need to think carefully about what you can do in a limited amount of time and with limited resources. But don't conclude that doing a qualitative study will be the easiest thing to do. Qualitative work does not require a big sample, but it requires extremely careful thinking and it is not easy to do well. So think, think, and think about what you want to do before beginning to write.

When you know what your purpose is, it is helpful to write the first chapter of the proposal while you are still working out your methods. If you have developed a clear rationale for your work, it is easier to figure out how to do what you want to do. Your committee chair may want to see Chapter I early, and may also want to see Chapter II if you follow the traditional format or our suggested new approach to Chapter II. Whether you use a traditional or new approach, every chapter should be as clear and as coherent as possible before you hand it in. So, when you have finished a first draft, don't send it off immediately; instead, wait a day or two, then look at it again and revise and edit before you send it to your chair. It is particularly important to make sure that your sentences are clear and grammatically correct: This shows that you are paying attention and editing, not just throwing something together and shipping it off. Remember that the more work you do before submitting materials, the less work you will have to do later.

While the chair is reviewing the opening chapter or chapters of the proposal, develop your methods, using the worksheet at the end of this book's Chapter 3 to help you think through issues and make notes for discussing them with the chair. You will probably need to revise the early chapters based on the chair's review. Work on developing methods as you revise, then send a draft of methods to the chair. Remember that once you and your chair are clear about methods, you may need to again revise early chapters to make them consistent with your plans. When you have a complete draft, it will go to the committee and you will get further suggestions. If some of these critiques seem contradictory or unclear, discuss them with your chair so that you can figure out the best way to resolve issues, and then rewrite again.

Indeed, writing a proposal involves rewriting and editing, again and again. For the dissertation, you do that under the supervision of your chair, but the process of revising, editing, revising again, and editing again is the same for any proposal you write, so think of this as one of the most important learning experiences of your doctoral program.

FIVE

NIH RESEARCH GRANT PROPOSALS

In this chapter, we address how to write National Institutes of Health (NIH) research grants, but please read this chapter even if you are doing a career development award or a fellowship proposal for the NIH, because each of these proposals includes a section in which you describe a research project.

SF424 (R&R) APPLICATION GUIDELINES

Once upon a time, the NIH used an application packet called Public Health Service 398 (PHS398). Applications were even prepared using typewriters! Then, some years ago, it was decided that the NIH should use the same application packet that all of the other federal agencies do (the SF424), but none of the applications were quite right, so the SF424 was adapted and some of the PHS398 elements were embedded within it, and the SF424 (R&R) was born (R&R stands for "research and related"). All of the NIH proposals we discuss in this book use versions of the SF424 (R&R). Please note that: (a) the (R&R) form of the SF424 is different from other SF424s, such as those used for HRSA proposals, though all SF424s are designed to have some similar forms, and (b) the PHS 398 elements that are embedded within the SF424 (R&R) are not quite the same as those in the old PHS398, for those too have been updated.

You can access the SF424 (R&R) guidelines on the NIH website (www.nih.gov); click on "Grants & Funding" and then (on the left-hand side) "Forms & Applications," and then "SF424 (R&R)." As of this writing, Version C is what you want to use, but this is sure to be updated in the future so always check to find the latest form of the guidelines before writing your proposal. The main version of the SF424 (R&R) (the first one on the list) is the one you want to use for "R" and "K" applications. What do "R" and "K" mean? R stands for "research," and the NIH offers several varieties: the R03 is for small grants; the R15 is for the academic research enhancement awards (AREAs); the R21 is for exploratory/developmental projects; the R01 is usually for larger projects (such as a full test of the efficacy of an intervention); and so on. K stands for "career development," and again, the NIH offers several options; for example, the K01 is for the mentored research scientist development award, and the K23 is for the mentored patient-oriented research career development award (you can learn more about preparing applications for the K01 and K23 awards in Chapter 6). There are many more Rs and Ks (and even other letters such as "P"): You can check them out by going to the NIH website and clicking on "Grants and Funding" and then clicking on "Types of Grant Programs" in the left-hand column. You will see lots of good information on each type of grant program.

When you go to the SF424 (R&R) page, scroll down and you will notice that there are separate guidelines for "F" awards—individual fellowships such as the F31 for predoctoral fellowships and the F32 for postdoctoral fellowships (Chapter 7 presents more about these fellowship applications). These also use a Version C of the SF424 (R&R) but be sure to check for updates and use the correct guidelines when preparing your proposal.

Keep scrolling down on the SF424 (R&R) page and you will notice at least two important things: (a) Supplemental Grant Application Instructions for All Competing Applications and Progress Reports, and (b) a section called "Additional Format Pages." Regarding the supplemental instructions: The SF424 (R&R) used to have three parts, but the SF424 (R&R) itself now contains only Part I—Instructions for Preparing and Submitting an Application. The earlier Parts II (Human Subjects) and III (Policies, etc.) have been combined and moved to a separate document titled Supplemental Grant Application Instructions for All Competing Applications and Progress Reports, which you can readily click on. Regarding the additional format pages: We talk about the ones you need, such as the Biographical Sketch and Planned Enrollment Report, in other chapters of this book.

Structure

What does an NIH research grant look like? The structure presented in Table 5.1 shows the most salient points of most NIH research grant applications using the SF424 (R&R). You will need a title, an abstract, and a project narrative, which is a few sentences that describe your project in lay language for use with legislators and others. Surprisingly, the research

TABLE 5.1 Selected Components of the NIH SF424 (R&R) Research Application

Title (200 characters and spaces maximum)

Summary
    a. Abstract (30 lines maximum)
    b. Project Narrative (2–3 sentences)

Research
   1. Introduction to Application (Resubmission Applications Only)— (1 page maximum)
   2. Specific Aims (1 page maximum)
   3. Research Strategy (12 pages maximum for R01, R15, R34; 6 pages maximum for R03, R21)
       (a) Significance
       (b) Innovation
       (c) Approach
       (Include Preliminary Studies where most appropriate)
Human Subjects Sections
   5. Protection of Human Subjects
   6. Inclusion of Women and Minorities
       (Planned Enrollment Report)
   7. Inclusion of Children
Other Research Plan Sections
   8. Vertebrate Animals
   9. Select Agent Research
  10. Multiple PD/PI Leadership Plan
  11. Consortium/Contractual Arrangements
  12. Letters of Support (consultants, consortial)
  13. Resource Sharing Plan (sometimes)
Other
  14. Appendix

Biosketches
    a. Research Team Members
    b. Consultants

Budget
    a. SF424 R&R Budget—Full or Modular
    b. Budget Justification

And so on
    a. Bibliography and References Cited
    b. Facilities and Other Resources
    c. Equipment

Notes: Not all components are listed—just the major ones --from the SF424 (R&R); the Funding Opportunity Announcement (FOA) always takes precedence. The structure of F (National Research Service Award [NRSA]) fellowships is discussed in Chapter 7 and the structure of K (career development) awards is discussed in Chapter 6.
PD, program director; PI, principal investigator.

plan itself does not take up a huge portion of the application. If you are resubmitting an application, you are allowed a one-page Introduction section to respond to reviewers' feedback on your last submission (be sure to read our advice on this and other sections throughout this book). If you are not resubmitting an application, leave this section out entirely. Begin the text of your research application with a one-page Specific Aims section and follow this with either a 6- or 12-page Research Strategy section, which includes the Significance, Innovation, and Approach sections (with your preliminary work put wherever it makes the most sense). People who are submitting small (R03) or exploratory/developmental (R21) research grants are allowed up to six pages for the Research Strategy section; those submitting larger (R01) or the AREA (R15) applications are allowed 12 pages for the Research Strategy section. Either way, as you can see, you must be concise in presenting your proposed research!

You can also see that there are lots of other sections that the NIH requires—Protection of Human Subjects, Vertebrate Animals, Bibliography and References Cited, Facilities and Other Resources, and so on. Fear not, for we discuss in this book all the sections needed.

Required Minutiae

NIH applications must be prepared using single spacing. You may want to double space drafts of the proposal so your readers have room to write, but before finalizing, you must convert the proposal into single spacing. By single spacing, the NIH means no more than six lines per inch. This does not mean eight lines per inch, and it does not mean seven lines per inch. Six means six! The fonts you are allowed to use are Arial, Helvetica, Palatino Linotype, and Georgia—so choose one of these early in the writing process and stick with it. The font size should be 11 or larger, and no more than 15 characters per inch are allowed in the text. However, tables and figures may use a smaller font size. When we say "smaller," please remember that some, or perhaps many, of your reviewers will be middle aged and if they choose to print your application and then cannot read the tables or figures without a magnifying glass, you are in trouble! The smaller fonts must still be legible. The NIH also requires that type be black and in the fonts allowed. In general, the NIH recommends that you stick to a one-column format and that you use at least one-half-inch margins all the way around the page with nothing in those margins (because the application packet will add page numbers and headers and such).

What about those pesky page limits the NIH specifies—do I have to follow them? Yes! What if I go over by just a portion of a page, certainly that will be okay, would it not? No! Do not do it! You must get your application into the page limits that are specified for particular sections. You are not allowed to use space you did not use, for example, in Specific Aims in the Research Strategy section. Why not? Each section of the proposal is uploaded as a separate file, and that portion of a page is lost to you if you do not use it in the section in which it is allowed. What if your text is shorter than the allowed page limits? Well that is okay, and reviewers will love you *if* you covered everything that was necessary. If you have left out important information, they may ask why you did not use the available pages to present that information.

Review Criteria (Briefly)

Before starting to write an application, it is helpful to know what reviewers will be looking for so you can be thinking about the readers as you write. If this cripples you, do not do it when you write—do it after you have a draft, when you are reading and editing yourself. The review process is discussed in more detail in Chapter 15, but let us overview what reviewers will be looking for in most research grants. There are five main review criteria, and you need to know what they are so that you can keep them always in mind. As laid out in Table 5.2, they are Significance, Investigators, Innovation, Approach, and Environment. Is the problem you are addressing one of significance? If not, or if you cannot successfully make the case that it is, why would the NIH devote precious resources to your project? Are the investigators the right folks to oversee and conduct the project? Do they (collectively) have the skills to do so and have they demonstrated that they can work together? Is there something innovative about the study—perhaps a new intervention or a new way to look at the problem? If, for example, you are studying the same old diet and exercise approach to reducing obesity, is there anything innovative that you are doing that would make it worthy of funding? What about the approach—have you designed and operationalized a study that can answer your research questions or test your hypotheses in a controlled and nonbiased manner? And is the environment a good one in which to do the study? Will it facilitate the work you propose? This is just a brief overview of what reviewers will be looking for. As described in Chapter 15, you can find additional detail under "Reviewer Resources" at the Center for Scientific Review (CSR) Institute's page on the NIH website.

WRITING THE NIH RESEARCH APPLICATION

The "guts" of a proposal are covered in the "Rationale" and the "Research Design and Methods" chapters of this book (Chapters 2 and 3). Here, we talk about how to write an NIH proposal using those chapters and following the structure of the NIH research proposal presented in Table 5.1.

TABLE 5.2 Primary Scored Criteria for NIH Review of Science

Overall Impact. Reviewers will provide an overall impact score to reflect their assessment of the likelihood for the project to exert a sustained, powerful influence on the research field(s) involved, in consideration of the following review criteria and additional review criteria (as applicable for the project proposed).

Scored Review Criteria. Reviewers will consider each of the review criteria below in the determination of scientific merit, and give a separate score for each. An application does not need to be strong in all categories to be judged likely to have major scientific impact. For example, a project that by its nature is not innovative may be essential to advance a field.

Significance. Does the project address an important problem or a critical barrier to progress in the field? If the aims of the project are achieved, how will scientific knowledge, technical capability, and/or clinical practice be improved? How will successful completion of the aims change the concepts, methods, technologies, treatments, services, or preventive interventions that drive this field?

Investigator(s). Are the PD(s)/PI(s), collaborators, and other researchers well suited to the project? If Early Stage Investigators or New Investigators, or if in the early stages of independent careers, do they have appropriate experience and training? If established, have they demonstrated an ongoing record of accomplishments that have advanced their field(s)? If the project is collaborative or multi-PD/PI, do the investigators have complementary and integrated expertise; are their leadership approach, governance, and organizational structure appropriate for the project?

Innovation. Does the application challenge and seek to shift current research or clinical practice paradigms by utilizing novel theoretical concepts, approaches or methodologies, instrumentation, or interventions? Are the concepts, approaches or methodologies, instrumentation, or interventions novel to one field of research or novel in a broad sense? Is a refinement, improvement, or new application of theoretical concepts, approaches, or methodologies, instrumentation, or interventions proposed?

Approach. Are the overall strategy, methodology, and analyses well-reasoned and appropriate to accomplish the specific aims of the project? Are potential problems, alternative strategies, and benchmarks for success presented? If the project is in the early stages of development, will the strategy establish feasibility and will particularly risky aspects be managed? If the project involves humans subjects and/or NIH-defined clinical research, are the plans to address (a) the protection of human subjects from research risks and (b) the inclusion (or exclusion) of individuals on the basis of sex/gender, race, and ethnicity, as well as the inclusion (or exclusion) of children, justified in terms of the scientific goals and research strategy proposed?

Environment. Will the scientific environment in which the work will be done contribute to the probability of success? Are the institutional support, equipment and other physical resources available to the investigators adequate for the project proposed? Will the project benefit from unique features of the scientific environment, subject populations, or collaborative arrangements?

Source: NIH (2013).

Introduction

The Introduction section is included *only* if you are resubmitting a previously submitted proposal and wish to have this proposal considered as a second submission of the same proposal. This section gives you one page to respond to the comments of the prior reviewers and to summarize the changes you have made to the proposal. This is covered in detail in Chapter 16, because you do not need to worry about it as you write your first submission.

Specific Aims

Perhaps the most important section of an NIH proposal is the one-page (single-spaced) Specific Aims: Every reviewer will read this section carefully to find out whether the proposed study looks important and new, and whether it has the potential for making an impact on health. Begin the section with one or two paragraphs that make the case for the study by showing the importance of the problem, the work done on the problem, and the need for further work. Conclude this argument by giving the purpose of your study. Then list your specific aims, followed by hypotheses and/or research questions. Finally, indicate what the next steps will be and say what the potential impact of this work is.

This is the first section in the proposal—but do not write it first. It is important to have a clear purpose and some aims before you begin writing the proposal (though the specific aims may change as you develop your methods and find out what will work and what will not), but you should write a draft of the Significance section (which comes next) before writing the beginning part of Specific Aims. The Significance section provides the rationale for the study; once you have a draft of that section, you can briefly summarize the rationale in Specific Aims. If you try to write Specific Aims first, you will waste time: It is a lot easier to summarize something you have already written than to compose a concise description of something you have not written and are not clear about.

The opening paragraph should present the problem: epidemic obesity, or the lack of continued breastfeeding for the recommended 6 months, or intimate partner violence, and so on. Show its importance in one sentence, giving figures on prevalence and severity, or providing other reasons why it matters. Do not waste any space on generalizations like "Diabetes is a major public health problem in the United States." Instead go straight to the data: "X millions of people are diagnosed with diabetes in the United States, and X have serious complications." Then zero in on the particular aspect of the problem that will be your focus. Will you look at the development of obesity in early childhood? Or dating violence as a precursor to partner violence? Will you focus on low rates of breastfeeding in a particular group of women? Briefly show why this particular focus or group is important. If we already know the importance of the overall problem—for example, diabetes, hypertension, obesity, cancers, and so forth—you may go straight to the aspect of the problem you will focus on; for example, the high prevalence of diabetes in Hispanics, or depression and anxiety in cancer survivors, and so forth.

Briefly summarize the research that has been done on the problem and indicate its shortcomings. This is the hardest part of Specific Aims to write: You need to both present the work to date and show why it has not gone far enough or why the interventions tested have not been successful—and you need to do that in very few words. To do this, first make a hard copy of the Significance section and identify the essential points on the research to date. Highlight those and then put them on another sheet, which will be the beginning draft of Specific Aims. However, when you begin work on this part of Specific Aims, do not write to space specifications. Most early drafts of anything are filled with flab—extra words, repetitious statements, explanations of the obvious, and descriptions of the irrelevant. If you try to write this part of Specific Aims in two paragraphs, your draft will still be filled with flab but you will leave out much of the meat of the section, so do not try to stay within a couple of paragraphs. Instead, say what you think needs to be said to make the case for your study. Your draft is likely to be closer to a page than two paragraphs, but then you cut and condense.

First, try to summarize the main points in just a few sentences; one sentence noting the extent of the research to date, the next describing the achievements to date, and the next summarizing the shortcomings of the work to date. Once you have a few summary sentences, look at what you have written and see if you have made a compelling case for a new study. The key is to make sure your logic is clear: Does your argument move from A to B to C? Or is it circular? Are there digressions? Have you left out part of the reasoning? Does what you have written accurately reflect what you are thinking?

The first attempt is not very likely to be compelling, so go back and see how you can strengthen your presentation, cutting out everything inessential and making your points sharper and clearer (always with references). The points you make here in Specific Aims must be the same points you make in Significance, in a longer version, but do not just copy sentences from Significance when you write Specific Aims. Readers like to think that you can make your case concisely, and they do not want to read the exact same thing twice.

Conclude this discussion with the overall purpose of your study: "therefore, the proposed study will do X." Follow the purpose with specific aims and hypotheses or research questions. We make numerous suggestions for stating these clearly in the next section of this chapter. It is important to remember that you have limited space, so if your purpose is really the same as the specific aims, you do not need to say everything twice: Either go straight to aims, omitting purpose, or omit aims and go straight from purpose to hypotheses and/or research questions.

Do not follow these with the proposed methods. You do not have space for methods here, and they should be summarized in the Abstract, which precedes this section. One caveat, however: In some basic science proposals, you need to briefly describe methods under each aim. Since experiment 1 will lead to experiment 2 and so on, readers need a sense of what experiment 1 will do in order to be able to see how it leads to experiment 2. Occasionally you will need to briefly describe methods in a more behavioral study—but only when methods are likely to differ from those that would be expected.

When you have delineated aims and hypotheses or questions, you need to conclude with a sentence saying what your next step will be. What will this study lead to? For example, if you are doing a pilot test of an intervention, the logical next step is to move to an R01 to more definitively test the intervention if this pilot shows beginning evidence of efficacy. And if this is a definitive test, the next step may be a study of ways to translate the intervention into broad practice. Always say what you plan next. Then conclude with a statement about the potential impact of the work. You might say that if this intervention proves efficacious and applicable to practice, it could make a significant difference in outcomes for those with heart failure. Or it could change the science of intervening by providing a new model that takes into account factors hitherto ignored. Be clear that these are not the outcomes you expect from the proposed study but potential outcomes of the work (or long-term expectations). If this is a basic science proposal, always tie the proposed study to a health problem or reviewers will not consider your work relevant for the NIH. Never neglect these last points. If you run out of space, delete something else.

Hypotheses and Research Questions

Typically, your aims are tied to your methods (i.e., operationalized) via hypotheses and/or research questions. This is where you get specific about what you are testing or looking for. If, however, you have research questions that do not add anything to the aims (i.e., if you find yourself just restating the aims) you can forego them—the aims statements are all you need. We would not recommend foregoing hypotheses, however—when they are relevant, they are needed.

Where do they go? They go right after the aims statements or integrated with them so you might have an aim, then the hypotheses and/or research questions related to that aim, then the next aim with its hypotheses and/or research questions, and so forth. Do not wait until a later section to state what your hypotheses and/or research questions are. Why? Because readers use them in addition to the aims statements to guide their reading. Some proposal writers wait until the analysis section to state their hypotheses, but we would not recommend that—it is too late in the process, and by then the reader is probably confused or has dreamed up a set of hypotheses for you.

Before going any further, it behooves us to mention that there are discipline differences about stating hypotheses or research questions. In some disciplines, proposal writers turn everything into hypotheses even if (in our eyes) it is premature to do so. Our recommendation is to use hypotheses when they are appropriate. When is that? First and foremost have the courage of your convictions. If you have just made a case for a certain set of outcomes in your argument, if you are testing the tenets of a theory, or if you are testing an intervention, you have expectations—capture them in one or more hypotheses! Second, the full test of a hypothesis will require several things: power to detect differences when they are there, pilot data to support the potential efficacy of what you are doing, and methods that are capable of soundly testing the hypotheses. When you have all of these things, you will probably want to state full hypotheses. Before that, you may have "working hypotheses," or perhaps you will be evaluating the feasibility of your intervention, or you may wish to obtain preliminary estimates of the efficacy of your intervention, or estimate effect sizes to guide your subsequent, fully powered study. Some of these (such as working hypotheses) may be stated as hypotheses without the word "significant" specified; some (such as estimating effect sizes) may be made sufficiently clear in the aims statement ("The aim of this study is to determine the effect size ..."), and some may require a research question in addition to the aim statement to allow more operationalization (such as determining feasibility: What do you mean by feasibility—do you wonder about recruitment? Retention? Attendance at the intervention sessions?) A research question might help you elaborate these dimensions.

A proposal is typically *not* the place to state null hypotheses. You will confuse the readers if you state that you "expect" *a*, *b*, and *c*, and then turn around and hypothesize that *a*, *b*, and *c* will not occur. Yes, you have taken basic statistics. Yes, you will probably be testing null hypotheses in the analytic procedures you use, but in the hypotheses you present here, state the alternative hypotheses—what you actually expect (and hope) will occur. The null hypotheses go unstated.

When you have hypotheses, how do you state them? At their core, hypotheses can be comparative if you have groups you are comparing, or relational if you have variables you are relating to one another. (Hypotheses may be much more complex than this simple comparative/relational focus, but these remain the core of your hypotheses.) Your study methods will help you determine how to state the hypotheses. In general, comparative hypotheses have the following elements:

- Who is being compared to whom
- On what
- When
- The outcome that is expected
- The expectation of significance (if the study is powered)
- How the variables are measured

What might this look like in hypothesis form? "It is hypothesized that women who receive the diet and exercise intervention will lose significantly more weight and have significantly greater decreases in their body mass index (BMI) preintervention to 3-months postintervention than women who do not receive the diet and exercise intervention." Note that the statement usually begins with something like "it is hypothesized that" and then goes on to specify all of the elements in the aforementioned list. If the statement becomes too complex when you try to insert how the variables are measured, you might want to add a second sentence to specify the measurement of the variables you discuss. "Height and weight will be measured preintervention and 3-months postintervention using a wall-mounted Health-o-Meter professional height rod and a Zeiss Digital Platform Scale, respectively. The National Heart Lung and Blood Institute's (NHLBI) formula for calculating BMI from height and weight will be used." Your Methods section will provide additional details about your approaches to measuring these variables.

An example of statements that do not quite make the grade as hypothesis statements might include: "Participants who receive the intervention will weigh less." When? In comparison to whom? Do you expect a greater weight loss in those with whom you intervene? If powered, do you expect the difference to be significant? As stated, a one-group-only design with a post-only assessment of weight is expected. Hopefully, your study is more evolved than that and has at least one control or comparison group with whom to compare those receiving the intervention. In addition, for most variables, the hope is that you have included both pre- and postintervention assessments so you can either compare the groups on magnitude of change or the postintervention scores, covarying out the preintervention values. (For some interventions, long-term follow-up is desirable, but if you are in the early stages of developing the intervention, you may need to hold off on examining the long-term maintenance of the intervention's efficacy.) If you are testing an intervention, you will probably wish to hypothesize a direction in your statement—for example, do you expect those in the intervention group to lose more weight than the control/comparison group? If appropriately powered, do you expect the difference to be significant?

Another example might be "Caregiving is burdensome for older caregivers." Uh-huh. But, can you elaborate the statement to operational-ize it more fully based on your study methods? Do you plan to compare older caregivers to younger ones? Do you expect the burden scores to be higher for the older caregivers? How is "older" determined? What about "caregiver"? How is the amount of burden measured? Your goal is to oper-ationalize your expectation(s) based on your study design and methods. Nothing should be a surprise to the reader—the hypotheses should flow from the preceding paragraphs.

For relational hypotheses, you typically will switch from focusing on between-group comparisons to relating variables. In general, relational hypotheses have the following elements:

- Which variable(s) will be related
- To which variable(s)
- In what direction
- When
- In whom
- Expectation of significance (if the study is powered)
- How the variables are measured

For example, "It is hypothesized that age and disease severity will be sig-nificantly positively related and social support will be significantly nega-tively related to level of pain at baseline in women with arthritis." Some may choose to state these same thoughts a bit differently: "It is hypothe-sized that the older and sicker the woman with arthritis is and the less social support she has, the greater her baseline pain level will be." Still others might state these as "predictors" instead of relationships (with age, disease severity, and social support predicting pain level), and that is fine—all of these are the same. As with the comparative hypotheses, a second sentence may be used to elaborate the measures of each of the key variables, with additional details provided about these measures in the Methods section.

The most important question you can ask yourself about each hypothesis, whether comparative or relational, is "Is it testable as I've stated it and given the design and methods of the study I propose to do?" Consider speaking with the statistician you will have on the project to make sure she or he has a way to test your hypotheses—*given the data you will be collecting.*

Research questions are often used when it is premature to posit hypotheses. Or they might be used when one wishes to delve into the data in more detail than the main hypotheses allow. Perhaps you want to explore the relationships of certain demographic or health dimensions to other variables. You might want to find out whether the intervention was more efficacious for some subjects than for others. Do you wish to examine a mediator or moderator that has not yet been explored by others so there is little literature to guide the development of a hypothesis? In these cases you would use research questions because your goal is more exploratory than it is when you have hypotheses. For example: "What is the relationship between social support and change in pain levels from baseline to 6-months postintervention in women with arthritis?" "Which women [based on age, education, and severity of disease] benefited most from the intervention?" "Will the effect of the intervention on pain, 6 months postintervention, be mediated by self-efficacy for pain management?"

In phrasing a research question, include the same types of information as specified previously for hypotheses, but typically you would not include the expectation of significance. As with hypotheses, your study design and methods help you determine how to state the research questions, and the research questions should go right here, along with the aims (and, if you have them, hypotheses).

Last, but not least, if you say that you have research questions, be sure to state what you are looking at as questions! It may sound silly, but often proposal writers will state that they are evaluating research questions and then present declarative statements, not questions. It is our hope that you will not do this.

Research Strategy

Significance

The Significance section is designed to show reviewers the importance of the study you are proposing. You do this by showing first that the problem matters and then by showing that you will do something about the problem that no one else has done. Thus, the Significance section makes the case for your study. We provided suggestions for developing the rationale for a study in Chapter 2, and we recommend following those suggestions. Here we add a few points specific to NIH proposals. First, you have to make your case fast. You have limited space for the Research Strategy, which includes Significance, Innovation, and Approach. With all that to cover, you cannot use more than two or three pages for Significance, and you should probably keep this section to a page for shorter proposals like the R03 and R21.

Do not waste precious space with general statements such as "Sickle cell anemia is a serious problem." You may need to begin with something like that to get started: It is a warm-up pitch; but later, cut out that sentence. You want the Significance section to begin sharply and to immediately arouse reviewers' interest. If you plan to intervene to help African Americans with sickle cell anemia deal more effectively with pain, begin like this: "X African Americans are diagnosed with sickle cell anemia, and every year they experience Y number of sickle cell crises causing extreme debilitating pain. Many go to emergency departments but are inadequately treated." Give reviewers data showing the problem is serious and needs attention, with references to back up your statements.

Next, tell reviewers what others have done about the problem. If your work is exploratory, describe what others have already found out about it; if you plan an intervention, describe the interventions already tried. First, report the general work in the area, using statements like this: "Numerous interventions have been developed to help individuals on dialysis deal with anxiety and depression," with references. Do not talk about every study individually: There is no space for that.

Then describe the interventions closest to what you propose, giving most detail on the studies you are building on. (Note: It is important to find out to whom your proposal might be sent and, if any members have done work in your area, include that work in your review if relevant.) Finally, point out why more work is needed, but do this with care. Be specific about what has not been done or what has not succeeded, because this is the reason for doing something more. But do not be overly critical of other researchers—they may be reviewers and you do not want to cause any unnecessary hostility on the part of your readers.

Conclude the Significance section by saying "Therefore the proposed study will do *X*," stating your purpose as in the Specific Aims section. This is the last piece of the argument for your study and you want it to be clear. Do not say something vague like "This study will fill the gap in the literature." You want to show reviewers that your work is what we need. If your proposed study is a basic science study, it is essential to tie the purpose to a health problem; do that here as well as in Specific Aims. Otherwise you will not be fundable by the NIH.

Next, if you have a conceptual framework, describe it here. The conceptual framework does not belong in Methods or in Innovation; it belongs here. Essentially you are telling reviewers: "This is our purpose, what we plan to achieve, and here is the reasoning behind our expectations." We made suggestions on conceptual frameworks in Chapter 2, and we recommend that you follow those here. But remember that the more physiological your work, the less likely you are to have a conceptual framework: Instead, you present the scientific reasoning for your proposed work. Basic science proposals never talk about conceptual frameworks. If your work is more behavioral, you may have a conceptual framework. Describe it briefly and make sure it matches your aims and hypotheses and your proposed methods. If you include a drawing, keep it simple and clear. Some institutes like a conceptual framework and they like to see a drawing, but if the drawing is not perfect, they will despise you.

One final note: When you do the first draft of the Significance section, do not write to space specifications. As we have suggested elsewhere, first write the argument that you think needs to be made to justify your study.

Then revise and revise until it is clear. Finally, go back and condense until you have a section that is both concise and compelling.

Innovation

The Innovation section is generally the shortest part of an NIH proposal and one of the most important: Innovation is one of the five criteria used by reviewers to evaluate your proposed study. The question you must answer here is: What is new about this work? While you need to show that for any kind of proposal, not just an NIH proposal, in most other proposals you describe what is new about your work as part of the rationale for the study. However, the NIH requires a special section in which you answer the question about innovation. The answer will, in part, determine whether you get funded. It is not hard for physiological researchers and basic scientists to answer this question: In such research you can say that you are developing a new method of preserving a transplant organ, are testing a new tool for rapidly diagnosing X, are developing a prototype of a new vaccine for Y, are developing a new way of analyzing the chemistry of A and B, or are synthesizing a new protein. The more basic the research, the easier it is to show that the work is innovative. The challenge for basic scientists is not to show that the work is new, but to make the connection with health problems: How will that new analysis of the chemistry of A and B lead to development of a drug for X? Or what does that protein have to do with colon cancer—what will it lead to?

With qualitative research, the newness of the work is also easy to show. For example, you might note that the research to date has clearly demonstrated that many people will die young from cystic fibrosis, but no one has asked teenagers with this condition about their personal experiences. Your study will do just that; clearly it is new. As with basic sciences proposals, the question here is, what are you going to do with the information to affect health? Develop a tool to assess other teenagers based on what you find? Develop an intervention to help them? Or what? What is the connection to solving this problem? Again, the link to a health problem is the issue, not the newness.

With more clinical or behavioral research, the link to a health problem is not difficult to show: Recognition of the problem obviously led directly to the study. The challenge here is to show that what you are doing about the problem takes others' work further, or offers a new solution to the problem or takes a new approach to a solution. Thus, to show innovation, you generally need to explain your approach. For example, others may have tested interventions for individuals to help them manage diabetes, but you are going to intervene with the whole family. Others may have developed interventions to help caregivers of family members with Alzheimer's disease, but you will be the first to help them when the family member has only recently been diagnosed—before the situation is dire. Others have tried interventions for hard-to-reach populations but without much success. You have taken a new approach: You worked with the community to design an intervention for this group and because it was developed with the community based on the needs of the community, it has a much better chance of success. The key is to show what is new in the approach; otherwise, no matter how often you say that your study is innovative, reviewers will conclude that you are not adding much to the science. Sometimes in a desperate attempt to find something that looks new in their work, researchers neglect their overall approach, which is what really matters, and instead focus on relatively trivial aspects—using a smartphone app to measure physical activity, or a new instrument to measure fall risk in the elderly. These may be new, but they are rarely the key aspects of your work, and they should not headline your innovation section unless they are your focus (e.g., if you are developing an instrument, the instrument is the innovation). Usually, what is new is the comprehensive approach you are proposing—to assess fall risk in the elderly or engage African American fathers in their children's development or help prostate cancer survivors deal with symptoms—so focus on that.

Describing this kind of innovation is difficult: You have to talk about the whole of your approach, not its parts, and show how that whole is new. Think about how you have conceptualized the study, and that may help you articulate what is new about it. The key here is thinking and carefully describing that thinking. You may also have some smaller innovations to point out, but do not focus on them. Do not go on and on about them. Sometimes your work will use an established approach but with a new population. In that case, presumably you have made a compelling case in the Significance section for studying or intervening with this new group. Then reviewers may conclude that the relative lack of innovation in the work is outweighed by the exceptional importance of working with this group. Generally, you should describe innovation in one or two paragraphs (though it may take more space for a basic science proposal). The challenge is to clearly present what is new without repeating the information about need that you just gave in the Significance section. It is helpful to first outline the points you want to make in this section. Do not begin by stating the study purpose; you said that at the end of Significance, only a paragraph earlier, and readers do not need to hear it again. And never begin by saying "This study is innovative because...." That is like saying, "Listen to me, this study is innovative; you have to believe me." Your job is to show, not tell. Begin with something like this: "This is the first study to do X or Y." Or "While numerous studies have tested in-person group interventions for X, this is the first study to use advanced technology to deliver such an intervention." Say what is new in the work and conclude with a statement about its potential impact (similar to the concluding statement in Specific Aims). You might, for example, point out that this study has the potential not only to improve self-management by people with diabetes but also to change the way we approach care and self-care of other chronic illnesses that bring similar challenges for patients; it may thus have a major impact on health. However, be careful; your work will have an impact only if it succeeds, so be sure to say that if found efficacious, this work may have such an impact.

Approach

This is the "guts" of your proposal. It is where you explain how you are going to conduct the study. If you are successful in explaining your methodological decisions, you may even be able to convince those with different opinions that you have taken a thoughtful approach to the problem at hand. Remember also that your proposal must make a coherent whole, so the methods you propose should flow from the earlier sections of the proposal.

If you are writing a research proposal, you will be proposing to do a research project or study. This is true even if you are proposing a career development award or a fellowship because these usually include a piece of research in addition to any training you propose. In these cases, the research provides an opportunity to be trained in research and lays the foundation for future research. For small research proposals, you typically are laying the foundation for larger studies to follow, but even if you are writing about a small research project, you need to think through and provide the details of what you propose to do. Needless to say, you *must* do this for larger research proposals—they require exquisite detail about all facets of the research. This section has different titles in different types of proposals. While some funders ask for "Research Design and Methods," the NIH asks for "Approach."

For most research proposals, you will want to start by reminding the reader of the overall purpose of your study and then include the following sections, when relevant:

- Preliminary Studies
- Design
- Setting
- Sample
- Intervention
- Control or Comparison Group
- Variables and Their Measurement
- Procedures
- Plans for Data Analysis

- Alternative Strategies
- Research Timeline

Let us begin.

Preliminary Studies. Most proposals for the NIH should include some description of preliminary work to provide evidence that the study you are proposing is feasible and likely to succeed. Preliminary work is not required for fellowship applications because you are a beginning researcher, but it is important in career development awards (though not necessarily titled as such) and for nearly all the R-level NIH grant proposals. If guidelines say preliminary work is not required, our advice is not to listen to that. Except for the small R03 grant proposals, every proposed study needs to be based on some initial work.

Preliminary Studies are usually, though not always, presented as part of the Approach section (they are allowed anywhere in the Research Strategy section). For clinical and behavioral studies, there are two basic ways to present this work. Before describing preliminary work, you can begin the Approach section with a brief overview of your study. For example, you might say that your study will test the efficacy of an intervention to increase completion of the vaccination series for human papillomavirus (HPV) by both adolescent boys and girls. Then describe your preliminary work. Or you can begin with preliminary work and give the overview after that. This decision depends on whether your overall study purpose is likely to be already clear to readers from what you have said in the Significance and Innovation sections, or whether readers need a little introduction to the study in order to see the relevance of the preliminary work.

If your major preliminary work has focused on some particular aspects of your study, you may want to wait and present this work with those aspects. If, for example, you have done initial work on an intervention or a measure, you may want to describe that work when you describe the intervention or the measure. However, if that work on the intervention or measure was part of a larger study or a funded study, you might want to give an overview of the big study in Preliminary Studies and add more detail in the relevant sections later in the proposal.

Begin the description of preliminary work with a brief overview of the qualifications of the research team, starting with the principal investigator (PI), then moving on to all major team members. Also, include consultants here, but do not include staff members. In this brief description of the team (no more than one long paragraph), the statement about each team member's expertise should be very short—no more than a clause or sentence. You do not have space for more than that, and besides, all the team members will describe their expertise in the personal statement on the first page of the biosketch they submit. So you do not need much here. The aim is to show reviewers that your team includes expertise and experience in all the areas needed for the study. For example, if your study is quantitative, you need to note that the team includes a statistician or biostatistician, or reviewers will not believe that you can handle the statistical analyses. If you or other team members have relevant clinical experience, note that also.

However, when you describe team members, do not say things like Dr. John Doe is associate professor of psychiatry at X university. That information will be on the biosketch and, further, it does not say anything about John Doe's expertise. You need to say that he is an expert in attention deficit hyperactivity disorder (ADHD) or schizophrenia or whatever the area is in which you need an expert. Only give the person's title if it indicates importance for the study. For example, if you plan to study brain tumors, it will be useful to say that co-investigator Dr. Sara Slow is director of the Brain Cancer Center at X Medical Center. Then add a sentence on her particular expertise; otherwise omit titles.

Do not say what team members' roles in the study will be. For example, you do not need to say that Dr. Nancy Flow will train the interventionists in the study protocol. That information belongs in the Budget Justification, where you explain what you are paying investigators to do. Only describe a role if it appears crucial for reviewers to know that now. However, do include statements showing that the team members have worked together. For example, have you published together? Collaborated on prior studies? Worked together on the pilot work for the proposed study? This information is important to show reviewers that you are in fact a team. Conclude the team description with a sentence saying that "Preliminary work for the proposed study is briefly described as follows."

As in other parts of a proposal, do not write this team description to space specifications on the first try. Instead, say what you think needs to be said to convey the expertise of the team, then cut back later. After you have written this section and the rest of the Preliminary Studies section, you will see what is essential and what can be cut.

Sometimes people describe the team after describing their preliminary work. Generally, we advise putting the team first because that sets the stage for the preliminary work. Also, you want the description of the preliminary work to lead directly to what you plan next—your proposed methods—and you break that flow by inserting the description of the team between the two. However, this is a judgment call. For example, if you have done some preliminary work but expanded your team and added new expertise, it may be important to put the team description after the preliminary work, emphasizing the new expertise.

The description of preliminary work should show that what you have done leads to what you propose and the proposed work is likely to succeed. Do not describe all of your previous research. You do not have space enough for that. For example, if you have conducted research that is related but does not directly lead to the proposed study, mention it in the team description, not here. Let's say you plan to look at the quality of pediatric palliative care; you might note in describing the team that the PI has done extensive research on children with childhood cancers; this shows that you know the area to be studied, but since the research is not directly related to palliative care, you do not describe it in detail.

Reviewers do not want a description of the study that led to the study that led to the study that finally led to what you are proposing, so stick to the last one or two studies—those that directly lead to the proposed work. If a co-investigator has done a study that is crucial to what you plan, include that here. But always describe the PI's work first.

Begin the description of each preliminary study by giving the title of the study, dates of the study, the PI, your role if not PI, and funding and funding source, with a grant number if there is one. Then describe the study as if you were writing a brief report or abstract. Do not simply mention the study and then talk about how useful it has been: Reviewers will have no idea why it is useful if you do not tell them what you did and how it turned out. Generally, you do not need headings like Purpose, Methods, and Findings, but that depends on the length of your description: The longer the report, the more helpful it is to have headings. With or without headings, it is important to first give the study purpose and briefly describe the methods. If this was an intervention study, it is particularly important to tell reviewers how the intervention was done and how its efficacy was measured. Then concentrate on the findings. This is the most important information for reviewers since this is what you are building on. Remember that you are using this prior work to help make the case for the study you are proposing.

Be clear about the number of people you expected for your sample, the number you actually obtained, and any attrition of participants. If you failed to recruit the sample you needed or you had high attrition, you cannot just say next time we hope it will be better. You need a convincing explanation for why that will not happen again: This time you will get the number of participants you need—and keep them. Also, if you did not get the people you were most interested in, explain that and provide a plan for ensuring that these people will participate in the next study. If you found that some measures did not function well with your sample, explain why and indicate what you will do differently in the next study. For example, you may have found that a measure of quality of life translated into another language was semantically equivalent—the words all meant the same thing—but the concepts measured were not relevant to the participants. So you did not find out what you wanted to know.

If you have done pilot work on an intervention, it is important to describe the outcomes. If, for example, your intervention was designed to help older women manage their diabetes better, and you operationalized that as improving exercise, diet, foot care, and self-monitoring of blood sugar, you need to say whether their self-management improved in all these aspects. If so, that provides a strong argument for the more definitive test you are proposing. But perhaps they improved in some aspects and not others. You need to offer an explanation for that and note that in order to deal with this issue, in the proposed study you will add more information or support for whatever came up short—daily monitoring or exercise or weight loss, and so on.

If you compared the intervention group to a control or comparison group, did you have a big enough sample to test your hypotheses? If so, were they supported? You probably will want to include tables or figures showing the data. If the hypotheses were supported, that is great, but you will need to explain why a further study is needed. Perhaps, you had enough participants to test some hypotheses but not others, or perhaps you are changing the study in some ways, adding another intervention or a booster, and so on. What if the intervention group improved, but your control group also improved and thus there were no significant differences between them? If that is the case, you must explain why you think the intervention is efficacious enough to be worth testing again.

Conclude the description of each study by listing any publications from the study, including those in press. You can also mention articles under review though they will not be in your biosketch. Finally, include a sentence or two showing how you are building on this work and, as noted previously, any methodological changes you are making to strengthen the work.

For basic science proposals, there are two ways to present preliminary work. Many researchers present the preliminary work for each experiment they propose just before describing the experiment. Thus, preliminary work is spread throughout the Approach section. If, for example, you are proposing a series of experiments to determine the role of genetics in the development of a particular cancer, you may describe what you have already done under the heading for each experiment. Often these experiments are presented under specific aims, so you begin your Approach with Aim 1, describe the preliminary work, describe the proposed experiment, then move on to Aim 2. However, some researchers describe all the preliminary work first, then present what they are proposing. Again, this is a judgment call: If the prior work will be clear if you present all your prior experiments together, either chronologically or logically, do so; if not, present prior experiments in conjunction with your proposed experiments. Conclude the Preliminary Studies section with a general statement noting how this prior work provides the foundation for the proposed study.

Design. We recommend that you begin your research plan with a statement about the design of your study (preceded by a heading that reads "Design"). This is not just a jargon-filled statement merely labeling the design. For example, the statement that this study will use a "quasi-experimental, repeated-measures design" may tell the reader that you have learned the jargon for what a design is called, but it says very little about what the actual study design will be. Why? Because many different designs fit that label. So name it, but then go on to say what you mean by that label—how you are operationalizing it in this situation. Describe the design in English by saying what you are going to do to whom, and when and what you will measure on whom. For example, you might have a design statement such as this: "The proposed study will use a randomized two-group, repeated measures design with one group receiving the experimental social support intervention and usual care and one group receiving only usual care. The intervention will consist of six contacts over 6 weeks. Data on caregiver burden will be collected at three time points: at Week 1 prior to random assignment (T1-baseline), at Week 6 when the intervention has been completed (T2-postintervention), and at Week 12, 6 weeks after completion of the intervention (T3-follow-up)." Note that the design statement is brief and the design has been labeled, but it is also described for the reader. You do not need to go into detail about how the intervention will be delivered or how you will measure key variables, because these will be described in their respective sections. But *do* provide readers with a roadmap to guide their understanding of the sections that will follow. This is an "overview" of what the study will be. If, by chance, you will conduct the research in several phases, you might consider overviewing those phases here, and then presenting each phase in its entirety, beginning each section with "Phase No. X," followed by the design of that phase. Or if you are doing a secondary analysis of an existing dataset, tell us briefly what the original design was before moving on to your proposed study design. Context is needed.

When the design is complex, it may help the reader to see a graphic depiction of it, but if the graphic depiction simply repeats what is in the text, it does not really add anything and just takes up space, so do not include it. Two examples of designs that might be helped by having graphic depictions are included here. In the first (Table 5.3), the researcher has used the Xs and Os that are taught in most research courses. There are three groups in this study. Twelve weekly intervention sessions will be delivered during Weeks 2 to 13 to the Intervention and Intervention + Booster groups, and 7 weekly phone boosters will be delivered only to the Intervention + Booster group during Weeks 15 to 21. Observations will be made on subjects in all groups in Weeks 1, 14, 22, and 26. Specifications of the "T1," and

TABLE 5.3 Study Design Diagram 1

Group	Week 1 T1	Weeks 2–13 Intervention	Week 14 T2	Weeks 15–21 Booster	Week 22 T3	Week 26 T4
			Study Week			
Intervention	O	X_1	O		O	O
Intervention + Booster	O	X_1	O	X_2	O	O
Usual Care	O		O		O	O

O, observation; X_1, weekly, in-person intervention; X_2, weekly phone booster.

so on, times of measurement are included so that the table matches what the researcher is saying in the text, and the footnotes help explain what is in the figure. It would be rather difficult to capture all of this detail in text alone, but you might be able to.

Another researcher might choose to include a design graphic because the study is measuring a number of variables at multiple times during a 24-hour period, and it will help the reader to visualize what the researcher is doing (Table 5.4). Note that this researcher has chosen to use Xs instead of Os for the observations, but this is okay as long as you use one approach consistently and make it clear to the reader. As you can see, this researcher will have quite a lot to talk about in the measurement section. For each figure you use to elaborate your design, be sure to include some text so it does not seem like the design figure is just plopped into the proposal; it takes text (and sometimes the figure) to describe your design.

For basic science proposals, you may find it most logical to describe your methods in relation to particular specific aims. In that case you might begin the Research Design and Methods section with a sentence saying that methods will be discussed under the appropriate aims, then relist Specific Aim 1, give the reasoning for the proposed experiment, drawing on your preliminary work as well as the work of others, and describe your design for the first experiment, thus: "We will determine the effect of X on Y in 12- and 24-week-old mice in the presence and absence of Z." Here you can say where you will obtain the animals and how they will be cared for; and if they will generally be cared for in the same way, note that, or you can hold that information until you get to the Sample section for your first experiment. Next describe in detail the experimental methods you will use for this aim. Follow a similar approach for other aims/experiments.

TABLE 5.4 Study Design Diagram 2

Variables	Afternoon	Evening	Sleep—Hours 1–4	Sleep—Hours 5–8	Early Morning	Late Morning
Pain	X	X			X	X
Perceived Somnolence	X	X			X	X
Blood Pressure (hourly)	X	X	X	X	X	X
Heart Rate Variability		X		X		
Sleep Quality (continuous)			X	X		
Perceived Sleep Quality					X	

X, measurement.

Setting. You will get your subjects from somewhere and you will do your study somewhere. These are called "settings" (or "sites"), and they need to be described. This is not the place to talk in generalities to protect identities of institutions as you do in published articles (e.g., a large southeastern hospital)—be specific, because readers need to be able to match letters of support in the application with what you say in the text (and, yes, you will need to obtain letters of support from your research settings—more later).

For *each* setting (or site) that you will use to obtain subjects, say what type of facility it is, where it is located, who it serves, and how many people it serves who are similar to the subjects you need; and include a letter from an appropriate individual (not just your best friend) providing access to the setting for your recruitment. Perhaps you will be recruiting premature babies and their parent(s) from a neonatal intensive care unit (NICU) within a larger facility. Quickly talk about the larger facility, then move on to specifics about the NICU. Perhaps the larger facility serves 35,000 patients a year—but that is not as relevant to your project as the number of premature babies served in the NICU. Where are these babies from—are they from the city or state in which the NICU is located, or perhaps from around the nation or the world? Are you only studying babies with heart valve problems? What percentage of the premature babies the facility serves has this problem—how many does it serve? And so on. As you can see, you will need to collect some data about each of your recruitment settings so you can present the relevant information in your proposal. In NIH proposals, you have several chances to do this: in the Setting section, in the letter(s) of support from the settings, and in the Facilities and Other Resources section (discussed later). To save space, in the text of the Setting section, you can provide some text along with a table that summarizes key characteristics of the settings you will be using to recruit subjects, then provide more detail in the Facilities and Other Resources section.

What if you are recruiting subjects directly from communities? You might want to let the reader know a little about these communities, often in a brief text and tabular presentation. For example, if you are putting up flyers in grocery stores throughout several communities—what are the communities like demographically? How many grocery stores? And which of their populace are you hoping to reach with this method? Are you recruiting from public health clinics in several communities? Who do they serve, and who do you hope to reach? Readers are going to review this information to decide whether you are likely to be able to access the individuals you are interested in (i.e., the recruitment settings will provide access to the needed subjects) and whether you have introduced any bias into the selection.

You may also have settings for the conduct of your research—where you will do the study. These settings might be where you are going to obtain informed consent, where you will conduct the intervention, and/ or where you might assess or measure folks (especially if these are all in different places). Some of the activities might be face-to-face, in a clinic, in a person's home, in a community location selected by the subject, and so forth. You do not need to describe the indescribable—for example, you do not know what each person's home will be like, but you might have conditions you will impose: The setting must be no more than x miles or y minutes from your research site, you will ask other family members who may be present to relocate to a different room, and so forth. Think it through and describe all the relevant settings as best you can.

If you are using more than one setting to recruit subjects, the comparability of the settings is very important, particularly if you are going to evaluate an intervention that will be undertaken in multiple settings. Readers will want to know whether conditions in the settings are comparable, so present the information needed to enable readers to compare them and, if you believe the settings to be comparable, make a case for that. Do they serve similar types of patients? Do they follow similar protocols?

Are their outcomes similar? If they are not similar, do you have good reasons for using these settings? Are you perhaps trying to access a broad and comprehensive population? If so, explain your rationale to the reader and indicate what information you will collect (perhaps about the setting, about the care received, about other services sought) to document exactly what is going on at each setting and to enable you to control these dimensions in the analysis.

What if you are using an electronic format to intervene or collect data? You may not have the level of setting description mentioned previously, but think about your subjects—how will they access the electronic material? Perhaps you will expect them to have computers at home (be sure to document the percentage who do!), or they may take their laptop computers or tablets to a community wi-fi setting, or they may go to a library. In these cases, you have settings to describe. This is also true if you are calling people on the phone—are there any setting restrictions and, thus, descriptions to provide? If so, do so.

Sample. The next section is Sample, and it is an important one. There is a lot to cover, and it behooves you to think through the issues carefully. You might want to keep a notebook on all of the methods decisions you have made to help you write the Approach or Research Design and Methods section, and nowhere is that more important than for the Sample section. It is easy to forget why you decided what you did, but if you keep notes of what the alternatives were, what you decided, and why, life will be easier.

The Sample section is likely to include a number of topics, such as:

- The persons you will be studying and the inclusion/exclusion criteria for those subjects
- The way subjects will be selected
- The number of subjects you will study and the way that number is determined
- Anticipated attrition
- Flow of subjects through the study
- The way subjects will be assigned to groups (if relevant)
- Recruitment plans
- Minority recruitment plans
- Retention plans

There may be other topics that are relevant for you, but let us address these first.

The persons you will be studying and inclusion/exclusion criteria for those subjects. Readers want to know whom you will be studying, because they want to be assured that you have appropriate plans to access the relevant individuals and that your plans will not introduce bias into the sampling. Whom will you be studying? Perhaps it is children with epilepsy, older-adult males with congestive heart failure, or female breast cancer survivors. In each case, specify whom you will be studying in general terms; then use the inclusion criteria to *define* the group and use the exclusion criteria for further *refinement* if needed. Let us first consider children with epilepsy. Inclusion criteria might include: (a) a particular age range of the children you will study, (b) a formal diagnosis of epilepsy, (c) epilepsy of a certain type or perhaps severity, (d) a requirement that the child has been living with the illness/diagnosis for at least a certain period of time, and so forth. The group might then be refined by excluding those who are too ill to respond to the study questions. You will quickly see that you need to specify *how* you will ensure that subjects meet your inclusion and exclusion criteria. Specify those methods right here in the Sample section. For example, perhaps the clinic from which you are recruiting subjects will agree only to give you the names of children who meet your inclusion criteria or perhaps you can screen for certain inclusion or exclusion criteria by asking questions of parents of potential child subjects (be sure the questions are appropriate for lay people). Perhaps you will obtain permission from the parent to query the child's doctor about certain medical criteria. Whatever your plans, they should be appropriate and reasonable, and you will want agreement from clinical facilities to be reflected in their letters of support.

Note also that the same dimensions should not be covered under *both* inclusion and exclusion criteria listings. If age is an inclusion factor (e.g., the child must be between the ages of 10 and 14), it is *not* also an exclusion factor (children younger than the age of 10 or older than the age of 14 will be excluded). You do not need both—it would be redundant. Do provide the rationale for any inclusion and exclusion criteria that might be questioned. For example, in this case, you have chosen the age range 10 to 14. Why? Your decision should have a scientific basis, not just a convenience basis. While we are talking about children, this is a good time to bring up the issue of exactly who your sample is. Perhaps your interest is in young children with epilepsy, but you know that the young children cannot provide the information you need, so you are going to ask a parent to complete your interviews or questionnaires about the child. In this case, the parent is also a subject, so be sure to specify this in your sample section.

Let's say you will study older adult males with congestive heart failure. After making this general statement, you might want to define each of the parameters via inclusion criteria: What do you mean by "older adult"? Specify the required minimum age (and perhaps a maximum). "Males" is pretty easy to determine—from medical records or merely asking the person. Should the person have a diagnosis of congestive heart failure? Do you require that he has lived with the illness/diagnosis for at least a specified period of time? What about severity? And so forth. For exclusion criteria, you might want to consider things such as whether the person is cognitively intact so that your interviews/questionnaires/intervention make sense. Also, is your instrumentation appropriate only for English-speaking individuals? And for all of these, how will you go about determining the things you need to know in order to include or exclude someone? For example, will you use something like the Mini-Mental State Examination (MMSE) to screen for cognitive ability? Describe how you will determine each criterion.

For female breast cancer survivors, the biggest thing to consider might be whom you are going to consider a "survivor." What do you mean by the word? Operationalize it via your inclusion and/or exclusion criteria, but whatever you say, it should not be a surprise to the reader. Prepare the reader for what you mean by survivor early in your proposal. Also, "breast cancer" includes lots of different types of cancers, so if you are restricting your study to certain types of breast cancer, specify what they are, why you have decided on certain types, and how you will determine that the person had that particular type.

Even though there may be separate sections later in the application which ask for information about the inclusion of women, minorities, and children in your study, we recommend that you include a bit of that information here as well. You probably will cover gender and age without even thinking about the fact that you have specified these dimensions, but ethnicity and race are also important to describe. You want the reader to get a good sense of who will be in your study. If ethnicity and/or race are at the forefront of what you are proposing, you will want to sample generously from the groups on which you are focusing. Be sure your recruitment settings can provide you sufficient access to the types of individuals you need, and describe ethnicity and race in both the Setting and Sample sections. Tables can be helpful in making a concise presentation.

The way subjects will be selected. Once the reader knows who you are going to study, your inclusion and exclusion criteria and how these will be determined, you need to specify how subjects will be selected. Remember, your method of identifying people should not introduce bias. Thus, you would probably not say that a physician will identify potential subjects and refer them to you—that method introduces too much chance of bias. Can you get access to clinic records or get a list of all of the individuals who meet your study criteria? Can you learn which ones have upcoming appointments if you hope to explain your study at their next clinic visit? Are you going to post flyers and have interested people call you to learn more about the study? If so, be sure you have a toll-free number that people can call, where they can either reach a live person or leave a voice mail 24/7.

If there are more potential subjects than you will need, how will you select among them? Remember, once again, you do not want to introduce bias. Will you take the first *n* people who indicate interest or who are available? Will you recruit a certain number at a time and finish with them before identifying additional folks? Usually, you will not randomly select individuals from the potential pool, because you will not have that luxury. It also is bad manners to get someone all excited about a study and then say, "Never mind, I don't need you." Therefore, think carefully about how you will identify and recruit the subjects you need.

The number of subjects you will study and how that number is determined. The *big* question that everyone asks is: "How many subjects do I need"? Readers will expect you to specify the number you anticipate studying along with a rationale for that number. If you are proposing a small exploratory or pilot study, your numbers may be smaller than for a larger, more definitive test of the efficacy of an intervention. Let's start with the larger studies first. If you are testing hypotheses (e.g., about the efficacy of an intervention or the relationships among variables), you will need a sample size that enables you to conduct those tests. Sample size is typically determined by using a power analysis, which is based on the paradigm of testing the null hypothesis. The needed sample size can be determined by specifying an alpha (Type I error), an anticipated effect size, and the minimum power. The alpha is typically set at something like .05 (1- or 2-tailed, depending on the hypothesis), the effect size comes from either the literature or your prior work, and the minimum power that is usually acceptable is about .80. Explain the details of your calculations for the power analysis. There are lots of programs and references out there to help you understand the process and calculate the numbers. The granddaddy of all of these is Cohen's book *Statistical Power Analysis for the Behavioral Sciences* (1988), but there are many other references, software packages and online resources. For larger studies, it is also wise to have a statistical collaborator/co-investigator so that she or he can calculate the desired sample size and make sure that the calculations are appropriate for testing the stated hypotheses. If you are not using the null-hypothesis testing paradigm, you will want to provide the details of how you determined the anticipated sample size and, hopefully, have a statistician on your team who is knowledgeable about the approach selected.

What if you are doing a more preliminary study—for example, pilot work to obtain estimates of the efficacy of an intervention or to determine its feasibility? In these cases, there is no "easy" answer such as a power analysis to guide your sample-size decision. You may want to think more about the *stability* of your estimates and the *variability* you need in the sample in order to answer your research questions. Think about your design. Each cell in the design must have sufficient numbers to enable you to obtain a stable estimate of what is going on and be large enough to capture all the types of people who might be in a study that will ultimately test your hypotheses.

What if you are proposing a qualitative study? Do not just avoid the sample size issue by saying that you cannot specify such things in advance. Estimate the anticipated sample size as best you can and describe how it might be adjusted during the conduct of the study. Be clear about the sampling principles you will be following, specify any relevant inclusion or exclusion criteria you will use, and cite references to support the decisions you have made. An "oldie but goodie" reference you may want to consult is Sandelowski's article on sample size in qualitative research (Sandelowski, 1995).

Anticipated attrition. If you will be studying people over time or time is involved at all in your study, you will need to think about attrition, estimate its magnitude, specify how you came by that estimate, and detail the plans you have to try to retain people in the study so that attrition is minimized. Let's say you are studying a very hard to retain group and anticipate that at least 50% will drop out along the way. Yikes! Perhaps the very people you are most interested in will leave the study, in which case the findings will not be generalizable. Or perhaps you do not have good plans to retain the control subjects who might not be getting a lot of value out of a study that takes place over an extended period of time; therefore, you anticipate a much greater attrition in this group than in the group who will receive your experimental intervention. Yikes again! The study groups are not likely to be comparable due to the differential attrition. These are just two of many possible problems. It behooves you, as the researcher, to think of ways you can retain individuals in your study so that groups are comparable and findings are generalizable (present this information in the Retention Plans section of Sample). Your goal should be to try to keep attrition as low as possible over the study period—to 10% to 20%. Be sure your estimate, whatever it is, is based on the literature or your prior work with similar subjects—and cite the source so the reader understands where you got it. Be sure, also, to include the anticipated attrition in your estimate when you specify the sample size you need. Thus, if the power analysis says you need 100 subjects and you anticipate a 17% attrition, describe your plan to oversample subjects to allow for the attrition ($x - 17\%x = 100$; $.83x = 100$; $x = 100/.83$; $x = 120.48$; since you cannot have part of a subject [.48], you will want to round this result to a whole number). (Note that you do *not* add 17 to 100: $117 - 17\% = 97.11$, not 100, and no, it is not close enough.)

Flow of subjects through the study. No matter what sort of study you are proposing, you will want to be sure that your settings can provide the sample you need to meet your goals—you do not want to propose something that you cannot successfully do, and you do not want your annual or final report to read "Oops—I thought I could get the sample but I could not," unless circumstances beyond your control interfere with your plans. Scientists have come up with a variety of ways to report actual sample sizes due to methods or other circumstances. The American Psychological Association (APA) tends to refer to these as "flow of subjects" (or participants) through, perhaps, a clinical trial or a survey study (APA, 2009). Others may call them CONSORT (Consolidating Standards of Reporting Trials) diagrams (www.consort-statement.org/consort-statement/flow-diagram) or something else entirely. Figure 5.1 shows a clinical trials version of a CONSORT diagram; many versions are available on the web so you can see how others have chosen to operationalize the CONSORT diagrams for studies (see pictures of CONSORT diagrams for observational studies and clinical trials here: www.google.com/search?q=consort+diagram&ie=utf8& oe=utf-8&aq=t&rls=org.mozilla:en-US:official&client=firefox-a&channel=sb); there are even diagram generators if you wish to use them (www.depts. washington.edu/hrtk/CSD).

We recommend that you estimate sample size *prior* to submitting your proposal (so you know what to expect) and put this information into the proposal so readers can see that you have thought through the anticipated impact of reality and your methodological decisions. For example:

1. For each of your settings, what number of subjects do you anticipate it will provide during the period you have specified for recruitment?
2. Of those, what percent do you anticipate will meet your inclusion/ exclusion criteria?
3. What percent will you approach/recruit?
4. What percent are likely to agree?
5. What percent do you anticipate will qualify for the study once fully screened?
6. If there is a time factor, what percent do you anticipate attrition to be?
7. And, finally, what number of subjects do you anticipate will complete the study?

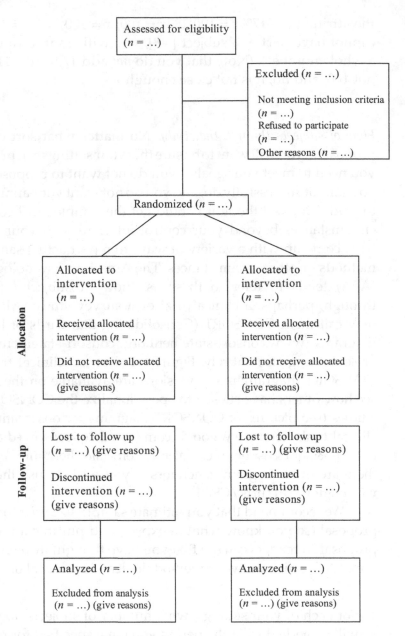

FIGURE 5.1 Flow or CONSORT diagram
Source: American College of Emergency Physicians (ACEP; 2008).

Let's go back to the example in which the power analysis and attrition estimates indicated that we would need about 120 subjects (perhaps 60 assigned to each of two groups). The clinical site you are using estimates that it can provide 20 subjects per month for the 6 months during which you hope to recruit subjects (thus, 120 subjects). Therefore, you are good to go, right? Not so fast! You have answered the first question, but let us go through the rest. Of the 120 the site can provide, what percent do you anticipate will meet the initial inclusion/exclusion criteria? Maybe almost all of them will, so let us say 90%. Ninety percent of 120 is 108. Will you be recruiting all day every day, or perhaps something shy of that? Let us say you are able to recruit 4 days of the 5-day work week, or 80% of the time. Therefore, your anticipated number from this site has just been reduced to 80% of 108 or 86.4. Probably not everyone will agree to be in your study, especially if it will take an extended period of time. But let us say that you are persuasive, and 85% agree to be in the study. The number is now 85% of 86.4 or 73.44. Perhaps you have some additional screening you will do to be sure the subjects fully meet your inclusion or exclusion criteria. For example, perhaps you do an MMSE to make sure that the person who believes herself or himself to be cognitively intact actually is. Let us say 79% of the folks pass the MMSE. You now are anticipating that the one site can provide you with 58.02 subjects. Subtract estimated attrition (let us say 17% again), for a final estimate of 48.15 subjects from this particular site. You are not going to meet the demands of the study with this one site. Researchers usually consider one of three options: (a) adding comparable sites, (b) extending the recruitment period, or (c) beefing up the recruitment methods so the numbers can be enhanced. Use whatever methods you can, but be realistic. This "flow" or CONSORT sort of thinking can help you be realistic in determining whether you can get the sample you need from the sites you have and also convince the reviewers of your ability to do so. (By the way, if the flow diagram takes up too much space for you to present in your proposal, consider running it sideways [broadside] instead of down the page or showing your calculations in the text as we have done previously. In most proposals, figures can be in a smaller font than the text, but they still must be readable by the middle-age eyes of an experienced reviewer, so do not make them too small.)

The way subjects will be assigned to groups (if relevant). Once you have recruited subjects (identified them, explained the study, obtained their agreement and informed consent, etc.), if your study has groups to which you will assign subjects (such as experimental and control groups), you will need to specify how you will assign the subjects to groups in an unbiased way. Typically, this will be done randomly, perhaps with stratification, so no bias is introduced in the assignment. But many methods are possible, so describe how you will do the assignments. Remember, especially if you do not have a large sample, that the method you choose may guard against the introduction of bias, but it cannot ensure that the groups are comparable on key variables, so you will want to compare the groups on these variables in your analysis and control for differences if the variables are related to the outcome variables. (Describe this process in your Analysis section.)

Recruitment plans. You may have covered this in earlier parts of the Sample section, and if so, you do not need to repeat the information. But if you did not cover it earlier, tell the reader exactly how you will go about recruiting subjects. Will you be available in the clinic so you can approach people who arrive for appointments? Will you use flyers in community sites? Who will do the recruiting? If not you, and especially if more than one person will do the recruiting, what sort of experience and education will you require of recruiters, and what training will you provide so that all recruiters approach folks the same way and give the same information? Your goal is to standardize how people will be recruited and provide the details so readers will see that you are not introducing bias into the recruitment.

Minority recruitment plans. Saying that you will have minority subjects in your study does not ensure that you will indeed have them. You may have access to them and you will need to document that, but having access to a group is not equivalent to their agreeing to participate. Your recruitment procedures may make the study equally attractive to all potential subjects. Yet perhaps some possible subjects do not want to participate in research because of the stories they have heard about research or because of the terrible things that have happened in the past under the guise of research. Your goal in the proposal is to detail how you will approach all subjects in a neutral manner and make participation in the study equally attractive to all. Will your recruitment materials depict a diverse group of participants? Will you post flyers in places likely to be seen by all the different types of subjects you hope to have? Do your recruiters reflect the diversity of the subject pool? Is your team of co-investigators as diverse as the population you hope to study? If it is a community-based study, are members of the community involved in setting the path for the research? And so forth. Consider using all the approaches you can to make the study attractive to all the types of people you hope to study.

For more basic science proposals, you may not have a sample; this may be a lab study. Or you may have a sample of mice or rats or other animals. If you have animals, say what they will be, where you will obtain them, and how you will handle them. Then say what you will do with them for your first experiment. If you are doing several experiments with the animals, you can provide general information on obtaining and caring for the animals with the first experiment and say that you will follow the same animal husbandry procedures for other experiments. Or you can provide this information earlier, after your opening sentence in Design and Methods, saying that you will describe methods under the appropriate aims.

Retention plans. How do you propose to retain subjects in your study? People have proposed many things, and you might want to try a goodly number of them. Perhaps you will have incentives (comparable for all subjects) and/or you will keep in touch via greeting cards or newsletters, send reminders each time you will be getting together, send small gifts at appropriate intervals, have a phone number where subjects can contact you if they need to reschedule an appointment, and so on. It is important to remember that you do not want to bias the results with the strategies you use. If you have multiple study groups, whatever you use for one group, also use for the others. For example, if you have incentives, give them for completing the assessments rather than the intervention sessions so that you are not actually evaluating the effect of the intervention *plus* incentive (which is not likely to be possible when the intervention is implemented in the real world). Your goal is to document how you will retain subjects in all study groups and, thus, minimize attrition.

Intervention. This section is included in a proposal only if you are planning to study an intervention; otherwise, ignore it and its heading (do not put "Intervention" and then "not applicable" or anything similar). If you are evaluating an intervention, the details of the intervention go here, with the heading "Intervention." After the heading, especially if you have a rather lengthy Intervention section, it is wise to begin with a brief overview of the intervention to provide the reader with a small roadmap to follow. Why? Because lots of details will be included here. At a minimum, they will include:

- Principles on which the intervention is based
- Preliminary steps you have taken to develop the intervention
- Intervention design—including content, structure, magnitude, and delivery
- Maintenance and documentation of intervention integrity

Principles on which the intervention is based. Surely the intervention is based on something. It may be designed to test aspects of a theory; it may be guided by the conceptualization you have posited earlier; or perhaps you have uncovered the tenets that guide its design from the literature. It may be an intervention that someone else has tested, but you are adapting it to a different population or situation. Maybe you have asked the patients themselves what it is they would like in the way of information, support, and so on. There are many possible sources of interventions, but in a proposal it is your task to describe the underlying principles in a way that convinces reviewers that you have a well-thought-out intervention with the potential to solve the problem you have presented.

Preliminary steps you have taken to develop the intervention. If you are doing an early study, perhaps requesting small funding to develop an intervention, you may not have conducted prior studies of components of the intervention, but you should have done some thinking about the intervention. Put that thinking into writing; specify the steps you have gone through: Perhaps you have reviewed the literature to see what interventions are already available and none meets your needs; perhaps you developed the content and divided it into the number of sessions you think you will need; perhaps you had experts review the content and delivery components; or perhaps you have enhanced an existing intervention. Whatever it is you have done, describe it here.

If you are further along in the process and have developed an intervention and done preliminary testing of it (perhaps obtaining information about feasibility or preliminary estimates of its efficacy), you will have much to tell the reader about. Tell the reader the things mentioned in the previous paragraph and then go on to write about the study(ies) you have done to refine the intervention or begin to determine whether it works. Perhaps you have done some work on standardizing the delivery of the intervention or determining whether booster sessions are needed. Whatever you have done needs to be described. Please make sure you *have* done preliminary studies before applying for larger funding (such as an R01 from the NIH). Typically, reviewers do not want to devote large sums of money to untried interventions; they want some sort of empirical support for what is proposed.

Intervention design—including content, structure, magnitude, and delivery. What content will you deliver in the intervention and how will it be organized? Will you be telling subjects about how to read food labels accurately and helping them practice the skill? Will you show subjects new exercises and provide a venue for them to work out? Will you perhaps teach parents to care for infants who are dependent on a technological device? Whatever it is you propose to do, describe it for the reader. Some people choose to present intervention topics in a small table; others present them in narrative form. Whichever you choose should give an overview of the content that will be covered, topic by topic. And the content needs to be organized in a coherent manner for subjects. Perhaps you will have multiple components covered sequentially in one session, or perhaps you will need to have multiple sessions to cover everything. In any event, tell the reader how you have organized the content.

It is also critical to talk about the magnitude (dosage) of the intervention—how much of an intervention are you going to give people? You want the intervention to be strong enough to accomplish your goals, not so brief as to not even create a blip on subjects' radar, but not so lengthy as to be burdensome. You are looking for "just right" or "sufficient," and you will have some work to do to figure out what is just right or sufficient. To get a handle on this, you might collect information via a small study asking people like those with whom you will intervene what they would like. Or you might ask experts for their opinions. You might review other interventions that have been fully tested to see what was done in those cases. Or you might do all of these. No matter what you are proposing to do, the amount of it matters, and you need to describe that.

You should also think about the factors that might influence your intervention: Do people need time to practice what you are teaching? Does the content need to be divided into manageable units so participants do not get overwhelmed or exhausted? Is repetition important? And there might be special factors that affect the population in which you are interested: Do you need to consider literacy levels? What about language or cultural factors? Age? Read the literature and think carefully about the people to whom you hope to generalize—who are they and what do they need from an intervention?

Sometimes you will want to tailor the intervention to each individual or to specific groups. For example, you do not want subjects to be uninterested in your intervention because you are trying to teach them something they already know. If a pretest shows that a person with diabetes already knows how to monitor her or his sugar level but not how to do foot care, you may wish to focus on foot care with that person. Another person may show on the pretest that she or he knows about foot care, but not about monitoring sugar levels, so you will focus instead on monitoring sugar levels. Yet another person might need information in both areas. Lots of researchers are interested in tailoring interventions, but they sometimes forget that it is important to think about what the overall test of the outcomes will tell you, since not everyone is going to get the same intervention. If you choose tailoring, be sure your hypotheses and analyses are appropriate for what you are doing.

There are many other aspects of intervention delivery that are important to think about and cover in your proposal. What mode will you use? Will it be delivered in person, electronically, by phone, other means, or via a combination of modes? Is there a specific location you will use or require for the person (gym, library, living room of a home)? What about timing? And will it be offered to individuals or groups? Will you be offering boosters or follow-ups of some sort? Are these boosters built into the intervention, or will they be offered exclusively to one group so you can evaluate them separately? Think through all aspects of the proposed intervention and describe them in your proposal.

It is also important to think about who will be delivering the intervention—the intervener. Why does it matter? If you have a highly technical intervention that requires a certain educational background and lots of training, readers need to know this. They will evaluate not only *what* you are going to do, but *who* is going to do it. The skill set and background should match what is needed for the intervention. But there is a reality aspect as well. If you require highly trained individuals to deliver your intervention and they are unlikely to be available in the real world, will your intervention ever be used? It is not likely. What is often recommended is to first conduct the research needed to test the intervention provided by persons with the desired educational background. Then, if the intervention is efficacious under these ideal conditions, the next step might be to see whether it works when delivered by the care providers who are available for a particular population.

No matter who the interveners are, they need to be exquisitely trained. You do not just say "Go forth and intervene." You want to ensure that all of the people delivering the intervention do so in exactly the same manner. You need standardization, and you achieve this by (a) developing a protocol for them to follow; (b) providing the same training to all of them; (c) having them practice on one another and with people like those who will receive the intervention; and then (d) monitoring delivery of the intervention and refreshing delivery skills as needed. Monitoring can take the form of modest checklists that interveners complete after each intervention delivery. You can audio or video tape intervention sessions, with the person on the investigative team who is responsible for the intervention reviewing the checklists or tapes and holding regular discussion sessions with the interveners. You can avoid all this by having only one intervener—but then you will never know whether the effect you find is due to the intervention or the person delivering it. By the way, do not just say you will monitor delivery of the intervention and leave the reviewer hanging about what you will do if you find that something is out of whack. Tell the reader what you will do in the event that you find an intervener has strayed from the protocol. Retraining perhaps? And, if that does not work...?

Maintenance and documentation of intervention integrity. When you write up your findings for a scholarly or practice journal, it is going to be important to say not just what you planned to do, but what actually happened. Did all of your interveners deliver the required content? Were there any deviations? Did subjects attend all sessions, or did some of them skip some so they did not get all of the intervention? Did you offer makeup sessions? It is important to document what happens when you intervene, so plan to keep records and describe the plans here. This information can be brief, but you will want to consider mentioning the things you collect, such as the checklists that interveners complete of the content they deliver at each session, times when contacts were made, deviations from protocols, attendance logs, and makeup sessions. Basically, your goal is to describe how you will maintain and document the integrity of the intervention.

Control or Comparison Group. Many people forget to tell the reader what will happen to the control or comparison group. They just assume that the reader will know that the control group receives "usual care." But what is "usual care" in this situation? And are you going to give the control-group subjects some sort of "attention" so that this factor is not confounding the results of your intervention? Readers will not know unless you tell them.

This section is usually short since there is not much space, but do not forget to include it. This is especially important if you are planning to use a comparison group instead of a control group, because such groups often receive more attention than a standard control group, or perhaps they are an existing group of individuals who are to be compared with your intervention group. Describe them and consider measuring what these people (and your intervention folks) get from others that is relevant for your outcomes during the intervention period. (Do not forget to note in the Intervention section whether subjects in the intervention group will also continue to receive "usual care" in addition to the intervention you are testing.)

All basic science projects are essentially intervention projects, though you may or may not have a comparison group, depending on your experiments. Therefore, for each experiment you plan, describe in detail exactly what you are going to do. Depending on the type of preliminary work you have done, you may describe that work as a whole in a Preliminary Studies section before Design and Methods, or you may describe the preliminary work for a particular experiment just before describing the experiment. If your preliminary work provides a general basis for the experiments you plan, it may be best to describe that work all together. But if the preliminary work is specific to a particular experiment, it will probably be easier for readers if you describe your preliminary studies just before describing the experiment.

Also, after describing their proposed experimental methods, basic scientists generally indicate what they will measure to determine the success of the experiment, and they often indicate the expected outcomes of the experiment. They may also include a section titled Alternative Approaches, which describes other possible methods and tells reviewers why they have chosen one approach rather than another. Sometimes that section also notes that if the proposed methods are not successful, the researchers will try an alternative approach.

Variables and Their Measurement. In this section of your proposal, it is important to convey to the reviewer what you are planning to measure, how and when you will measure these things, and what the characteristics of the measures are. In the old days, this section seemed to go on and on and on. There is a lot that needs to be covered, but typically these days you will want to summarize all you can in a table or two and add text to clarify what is in the table—not repeat it. Begin with a paragraph that provides an overview of all the domains you will be assessing and when you will assess them and refer the reader to your table(s) (see Table 5.5), which should appear right after this paragraph.

As a reviewer, it is hard to make sense of what will be measured if the writer just lists all the measures, either in the text or a table. *Organize* the information for yourself and for the reader. First, organize by "domain"

TABLE 5.5 Sample Table of Variables and Their Measurement

| | | | Administration Timepoints | | |
| | | | T1 Baseline | T2 Immediate Posttest | T3 6-Month Posttest |
Variable	Instrument	Psychometrics			
Outcomes					
Depression	CESD-R[1]	xxx	X	X	X
	DSM-5[2]	xxx	X		X
Anxiety	STAI[3]				
	Trait	xxx	X		
	State	xxx	X	X	X
Mediators					
Self-efficacy	Self-Efficacy Scale[4]	xxx	X	X	X
Social Support	Emotional Support Scale[5]	xxx	X	X	X
Patient characteristics					
Age	Demographic Form	N/A	X		
Education	Demographic Form	N/A	X		

Note: 1–5 indicate that references should be included along with those in the text in your reference list; xxx, insert number.

or "variable" for which you have measures; then organize the variables into those that are the primary outcome variables, and if you have them, secondary outcome variables; variables that you are using as predictors; variables that are mediators, moderators, or covariates; intervention variables (if you did not put these in your Intervention section); cost variables, if you are assessing cost as an ancillary dimension; and purely descriptive variables. (Note that the screening variables you measure to see whether people qualify for your study are described in the Sample section and do not need to be repeated here.)

There are many types of measures, and all that you are using should be summarized in your table. They might include questionnaires or assessments you have identified from the literature that (a) are appropriate for the dimensions in which you are interested; (b) have established psychometrics (indices of reliability *and* validity); and (c) have been shown to be relevant for your particular population. If you have developed an instrument/questionnaire yourself, the reviewers will want to know how you know whether it is any good, so you will want to do some preliminary work on appropriateness and psychometrics before submitting a proposal that uses the instrument.

The questionnaires you identify should be fully explained, and a copy of each should be included in an appendix (if allowed). The table you present may not have room for everything you need to include, so use the accompanying text to more fully explain what you cannot squeeze into the table. For example, if there is only room in the table for an instrument's acronym, say what that acronym stands for in the text. Do you have room to include the reference for the instrument in the table? If not, put the reference in the text. What does the instrument measure and how does it do so—might you want an example item and response scale? How many items are there, and how is the instrument scored? Are you able to put the psychometrics in the table? If not, elaborate on them in the text, using only those that are relevant to your population. Also include information about any adaptations of the instrument you will be using, and specify any further evaluations you plan on doing with the instrument in the proposed study. Be sure to specify the times when the instrument will be administered, appropriateness for your population, and the order of instrument administration, especially if you are using measures that can affect one another.

Last, but certainly not least, tell the reader how long it takes to administer/complete each instrument; or, if you wish, you can provide this information at the end for all instruments that you will administer to subjects. If the instrumentation is overwhelming or burdensome, you will have problems keeping people in the study, so you will want to elaborate here or in the Procedures section about ways you will reduce the burden. Will you allow people breaks? Will you provide opportunities for them to divide the data collection into multiple episodes? If you allow this, do you have restrictions on how long a break can be taken between episodes? Remember, too, that it is important to be efficient in what you measure; only measure what you need to for the study—you are not on a fishing expedition.

Questionnaires are not the only way that variables are assessed. You might also have physiological measures, biological samples, observational approaches, open-ended questions, structured interviews, document reviews, and so forth. Each of these approaches has its own standards regarding what you should present in your proposal; each needs to be presented in the same order as presented in Table 5.5. Table 5.6 presents a sample of the information we recommend that you include (at a minimum).

In basic science proposals, you generally indicate the measures you will use after you describe a particular experiment, not in a separate section. So this section is not relevant for you. The following Procedures section is also not relevant for basic science proposals.

Procedures. Writing a procedures section is like telling the story of what will happen to each subject as she or he progresses through your study. You include everything from recruitment to informed consent, baseline data collection, assignment to groups, intervention contacts (if relevant), additional data collection contacts, time commitments (subject burden), incentives for participating in data collection, and retention contacts/ activities. If you are going to do regular training of interventionists or data collectors, or if you are going to monitor each subject's participation, you can discuss those things here. If you have people in a wait-listed control group who are going to get a version of the intervention after participating in the study, you might want to discuss their progress through the study here.

However, you may not need a Procedures section if you have covered all of the salient material elsewhere. Is recruitment detailed in the "recruitment" section? If so, there is usually no need (and no space) to repeat it here. Is informed consent mentioned earlier and covered in detail in the Human Subjects section? If so, it may not need to be here. Similarly, if delivery of the intervention, checking of intervention fidelity, standardization of delivery of the intervention, attendance and active participation in intervention sessions, and data collection procedures are covered elsewhere, you do not need to repeat that information here. Thus, the Procedures section is needed only if you have new information to present and have the space to do so.

Plans for Data Analysis. For many people, this is a difficult part of the proposal to write, so it is recommended that you consider adding a

TABLE 5.6 Measurement Characteristics to be Presented for Selected Instrumentation

Physiological	Biological	Observations	Open-Ended Questions	Interviews
Variables to be measured	Variables to be measured	Variables to be measured	Variables to be measured	Variables to be measured
What will be used to indicate each variable	What will be used to indicate each variable	What will be observed	What will be asked	What information you hope to elicit/obtain
How the measure will be obtained	How samples will be obtained	How it will be observed (directly? via video?)	How the participant will be asked to respond	What the details might be
When administered (and frequency & timeframe if relevant)	When administered	When observed	When asked	When interviewed
Equipment used (including manufacturer & location)	Equipment &/or supplies used to obtain samples	If video, details of equipment, setup, focus, etc.	If audiotaped, details of equipment, setup, etc.	If audiotaped, details of equipment, setup, etc.
Reliability/ training in using equipment	Reliability/ training in obtaining samples	Reliability/ training in observational methods	Reliability/ training in questioning method if done in person	Reliability/training in interview method
Data reduction techniques/ scoring (if relevant)	Handling of the samples	How will you turn the observations into measures of your variables? Will coding be involved?	How will you turn responses into measures of your variables? Will coding be involved?	What will you ask? e.g., minimally structured interview: Begin with a broad opened-ended question? Say so and state it. Interview shaped based on subject responses? Probes – specify if and what they are if they are to be used. Audiotape? Transcribe?

(continued)

TABLE 5.6 Measurement Characteristics to be Presented for Selected
Instrumentation *(continued)*

Physiological	Biological	Observations	Open-Ended Questions	Interviews
	Laboratory the samples will be sent to for analysis Laboratory name Laboratory's expertise in this type of analysis How samples transported to the lab	If coding: Who will code? Using what schema? Has the schema been used before? Provide citations & evidence of quality of schema Training in the use of coding schema Reliability of coders – between and within Reliability checks	If coding: Who will code? Based on what schema? (developed from all responses? Expert review of your schema? Allow multiple codes per person or e.g., code first response? If multiple codes, code as present/ absent? Training in coding system Reliability checks	How go about summarizing responses? Coding? If so, describe your approach
				Might these initial plans change? Specify basis of decisions for changing
Citations to support your approach	Citations to support your approach	Citations to support your approach	Citations to support your approach	Citations to support your approach

statistician with appropriate (and demonstrable) expertise to your team
so she or he can either write this section, along with the Power Analysis
section, or guide you in its development or revision. If you are writing a
short proposal, this section will also be short and to the point. If you are
writing a more involved proposal, you will carefully lay out the plans for
testing each hypothesis or answering each research question.

Usually, you begin by discussing the steps you will take to ensure that you are going to manage the data well. The quality of your data management is as important as any other part of the project. Remember, garbage in, garbage out. So data need to be very, very clean when you begin to analyze them. What do we mean by clean? That you can assure that what is in the dataset is actually what happened—that you have carefully handled data entry (perhaps by using software to create data entry screens or sheets and double checking all of the data, perhaps by having double entry by two different people and comparing the resulting datasets, or perhaps by comparing the dataset to the original forms); and that you have done range and distribution checks, making sure all missing values are truly missing and that they are coded as missing, outliers are identified and corrected, and the distribution of scores is as you anticipated (if, e.g., the printout says that you have 50 males when your study was of pregnant females, you know you have a problem). For short proposals, this information might be provided in one sentence; for longer proposals you will go into more detail.

The next section typically addresses any preliminary analyses you plan to do. Did you say in the Variables and Their Measurement section that you would do psychometric analyses of any of the instruments? If so, here is where you provide the details. (Strangely enough, many people say they will perform psychometric analyses of the instruments, but do not say what they will do if they identify problems.) Do you have groups in your project (e.g., intervention and control) that need to be compared on baseline characteristics or dropouts? Here is where you describe those comparisons and what you will do if you find differences (e.g., if the groups differ on baseline characteristics, will you examine the relationships between those variables and outcomes and then covary out the ones on which the groups differ and are related to the outcomes in your primary analysis?). This is also where you want to mention any analyses you will do to describe the final sample.

Then move on to detailing what you will do to test each hypothesis and/or answer each research question. For each one, it is helpful to readers if you restate or at least paraphrase the hypothesis or question so they will not have to keep going back to the front of the proposal to see what you are testing. Next, specify the variables that will be used in the particular analysis and which measurement points you are talking about (if there are multiple timepoints). Why? Because, for example, the way you have framed your study might mean that the main test of your hypothesis is changes observed from pretest to the immediate posttest, with subsequent follow-up timepoints addressed in other hypotheses or questions. Be specific. Then tell the reader what statistical approach will be used to test the hypothesis or question. You may use something as simple as a *t*-test or a correlation or as complex as causal modeling or time series analysis. Whatever you choose, the criterion by which it should be evaluated is its appropriateness—not how complex, or sexy, or current it is. Do not choose the most high-falutin' thing out there just because it is available; choose what is appropriate. Your goal is to convince the reviewers that you have selected the best (most appropriate) analytic approaches for your study. Reference citations typically are not needed unless you are proposing something that reviewers are unlikely to know. Lastly, add a discussion of any special issues that may affect this analysis. Will you be testing to see whether you meet the assumptions of the statistical test? Will you be including any covariates? Will you be making any corrections for multiple tests? If these types of things are relevant, be sure to mention them.

There are other approaches to data analysis that are perfectly acceptable (e.g., Bayesian analyses). Just have someone with appropriate and demonstrable expertise in the area on your team and describe what you plan to do instead of just naming it. You usually need to go the extra mile if you are using something that is out of the ordinary.

What about plopping a generic data analysis plan into your study? It usually does not work, so it would not be recommended.

What if you are doing a qualitative study? Everything mentioned previously still applies, but it might have different names. You *do* have to think about data management quality. If you did not put the coding information (data extraction) information in the Variables section, put it here. You might be exploring relationships via data matrices instead of via statistical tests. You will need to document the analytic process, verify interpretations, and be sure to reference the approach you are using. Use the standards in your field to make sure you are presenting a coherent and complete analysis.

For basic science proposals, it is important to include plans for statistical analyses of the data you collect. This is sometimes an area that basic scientists forget to include—but that can be dangerous. For each experiment you plan, say how many times you will repeat the experiment, and what analyses you will use to test the significance of the results. Make sure that you indicate whether you will have the power to test the significance of your results. If this is not your strength, by all means get a statistician to help you.

Alternative Strategies. As noted earlier, most basic science proposals include a section titled Alternative Approaches, after each experiment described. We recommend that in clinical and behavioral studies, you address alternative strategies you have considered along the way, but some agencies ask for this section to appear here, so in that case it would behoove you to have it. You might want to elaborate on alternative strategies that were only briefly discussed earlier, or you might want to think about broad issues that were not relevant for discussion earlier. What if there was an alternative design you could have chosen for the study but did not? You might want to explore that here. For example, rather than choosing to observe premature infants for 12 months, you might have chosen to observe them for 9 months because such a timeframe coincides with their development. Or, rather than having an attention control group, you have chosen a standard control group. Your reasons for doing so could be elaborated here. No matter what you do, do not shoot yourself in the foot by leaving the reviewer wondering why you did not choose one of the alternative strategies. Have good (scientific) reasons for choosing what you did, state them, and leave the reviewer with a positive taste in her or his mouth.

Timeline. Once you have elaborated your design and methods, it is important to show the reader the timeline for conducting these steps. This is a timeline specifically for the research you will be conducting—not for training or other activities. Since space is a very dear quantity, present this in as compressed a format as you can. Often, people only have room for a header, a touch of text, and then a brief figure that shows the activities to be performed by month or quarter of the study period. In the table (or text), include things like your start-up activities, subject recruitment, intervention delivery, data collection, data entry and analysis, and report/ article writing. An example is given in two formats—tabular (Table 5.7) and text (Table 5.8)—but whatever approach you use, you will want to personalize the timeline to your particular study. This will be the same for basic science proposals as for more clinical or behavioral proposals.

SUMMARY

As you can tell, this chapter (and book) assumes that you have the knowledge you need to design and operationalize the study of your research questions or hypotheses. This is a proposal writing book, not a research design and methods book. If you need additional content on research design and methods, refer to one of the many excellent texts that are available.

TABLE 5.7 Timeline Exhibit 1 (Text and Table)

Timeline

The figure depicts the activities that will occur over the 3 years of the proposed project in 3-month annual quarters.

Months:	1–3	4–6	7–9	10–12	13–15	16–18	19–21	22–24	25–27	28–30	31–33	34–36
Grant activities: Start-up activities	X											
Hiring of grant personnel	X											
Making final site arrangements	X											
Training												
Training of interveners	X											
Training of data collectors	X											
Reliability study		X	X									
Baseline data collection				X	X	X	X					
Interventions				X	X	X	X	X				
Posttest 1 data collection					X	X	X	X	X			
Posttest 2 data collection						X	X	X	X	X		
Data analysis							X	X	X	X	X	X
Report and article writing				X				X	X	X	X	X

TABLE 5.8 Timeline Exhibit 2 (Text Only)

Timeline	
Months 1–3	Grant personnel will be hired, final arrangements will be made with the clinical sites, and all study materials will be finalized and printed.
Months 4–6	All interveners and data collectors will complete the 4-week training program.
Months 6–9	The reliability study will be conducted.
Months 10–21	One hundred subjects (approximately 25 per quarter) will be recruited into the study and baseline data collection completed.
Months 10–24	The 10-week intervention will be conducted.
Months 13–27	Immediate posttest (Posttest 1) data will be collected.
Months 16–30	Three month follow-up (Posttest 2) data will be collected.
Months 19–36	Data analysis will begin with the completion of collection of the baseline data and continue through the end of the project. Major analyses and hypothesis testing will be performed in the final 6 months of the grant.
Months 10, 22, 36	Project reports will be written and submitted to the agency. Work on project articles will begin after collection and beginning analysis of baseline data have been completed.

REFERENCES

American College of Emergency Physicians. (2008). Retrieved from http://www
.acep.org/search.aspx?searchtext=consort%20diagram

American Psychological Association. (2009). *Publication manual of the American Psychological Association* (6th ed.). Washington, DC: American Psychological Association.

Cohen, J. (1988). *Statistical power analysis for the behavioral sciences* (2nd ed.). Hillsdale, NJ: Lawrence Erlbaum Associates.

National Institutes of Health. (August, 2013). Retrieved from http://grants.nih
.gov/grants/guide/pa-files/PA-13-302.html

Sandelowski, M. (1995). Sample size in qualitative research. *Research in Nursing & Health, 18,* 179–183.

SIX

FELLOWSHIP PROPOSALS

Many agencies offer fellowships to support pre- and/or postdoctoral studies and research. They include foundations such as the American Cancer Society (ACS), the American Heart Association (AHA), the Robert Wood Johnson (RWJ) Foundation, and the Hartford Foundation, as well as the federal government through the National Institutes of Health (NIH). Some of these agencies have a particular focus to their fellowships; for example, the ACS is interested in cancer-related topics, the AHA is interested in cardiovascular-related projects, and the RWJ Foundation offers a fellowship in health policy research. Some agencies offer their fellowships directly through educational institutions. However, the NIH allows perhaps the greatest diversity of topics via its many institutes and centers and offers fellowships for those early in their research careers as well as those further along in their careers. The NIH calls these Ruth L. Kirschstein National Research Service Awards (NRSAs) and uses an "F" (for fellowship) to denote the type of activity. In this chapter, we address the F31 (predoctoral NRSA) and F32 (postdoctoral NRSA).

NATIONAL RESEARCH SERVICE AWARDS

The structure of an NRSA is shown in Table 6.1; it was created from the SF424 (R&R) fellowship application guidelines. You will notice that this fellowship application, as are most fellowship applications, is focused on *you*, the applicant or candidate. The proposal addresses your planned research training during the award, your research experience, and your long-term/career goals. The funder is investing in *you*; to train you to be

TABLE 6.1 Selected Components of NIH NRSA Applications

Title (200 characters and spaces maximum)

Summary
   a. Abstract (30 lines maximum)
   b. Project Narrative (2–3 sentences)

Research Training (the Guts of the Science!)
   a. Introduction to Application (Resubmission Applications Only) (1 page maximum)
   b. Specific Aims (1 page maximum)
   c. Research Strategy (6 pages maximum)
      1. Significance
      2. Innovation (not requested for fellowships, unless specified in the FOA)
      3. Approach
         (Include Preliminary Studies [if any] in Research Strategy)
   d. Protection of Human Subjects
   e. Inclusion of Women and Minorities
      (Planned Enrollment Report)
   f. Inclusion of Children
   g. Resource Sharing Plan (sometimes)

Training
   a. Goals for Fellowship Training and Career (1 page maximum)
   b. Activities Planned Under This Award (1 page maximum)
   c. Doctoral Dissertation and Research Experience (2 pages maximum)
   d. Respective Contributions (1 page maximum)
   e. Selection of Sponsor and Institution (1 page maximum)
   f. Responsible Conduct of Research (1 page maximum)

Sponsor and Co-Sponsor Information (6 pages maximum)
   a. Research Support Available
   b. Sponsor's/Co-Sponsor's Previous Fellows/Trainees
   c. Training Plan, Environment, Research Facilities
   d. Number of Fellows/Trainees to Be Supervised During the Fellowship
   e. Applicant's Qualifications and Potential for a Research Career

Biosketches
   a. You
   b. Sponsor(s)

Etc.
   Vertebrate Animals
   Bibliography and References Cited
   Facilities & Other Resources
   Equipment
   Appendices
   List of Referees
   Letters of Reference (3-5 submitted separately)

Note: Content has been reorganized a bit and not all components are listed—just the major ones—from the SF424 (R&R); the Funding Opportunity Announcement [FOA] always takes precedence.

a scientist so you can make important contributions to the field for years to come. There is also a place for your sponsor(s)/mentor(s) to add their views and a place for ancillary materials. The goal of the fellowship is to enhance your "potential for, and commitment to, an independent scientific research career in a health-related field" (NIH, 2014, Overall impact/merit, para 1). Reviewers will focus on your *potential* for a productive career, your *need* for training, and the degree to which the proposed research training, the sponsor, and the environment will *satisfy those needs*. Please keep these things in mind as you consider writing a training proposal: Do you *need* it, or are you just proposing what you would do anyway? If the latter is true, why would they fund you? If you do not plan to *continue* in the research world as an independent investigator, why would they fund you? If you have not had any research experience so far, why would they believe that you will capitalize on the award by doing research in the future? (The scored review criteria for NIH pre- and postdoctoral fellowships are summarized in Table 6.2, and complete review criteria can be found at www .grants.nih.gov/grants/peer/critiques/f.htm.)

Research Training

Your proposed research goes in this section. Notice that it is called "research training" instead of "research." This is because your project is seen not only as a piece of research but also as an opportunity for you to learn about doing research. Reviewers expect most of the usual sections (Specific Aims, Research Strategy, and all of the ancillary materials, e.g., about human subjects or, if you will use them, vertebrate animals). You can find these topics covered in this book in Chapters 5 and 13. The NIH indicates that the Innovation section in Research Strategy is not required for NRSA applications; however, while it is not required, we encourage you to read what we have to say on the topic (in Chapter 5) and, *if* you have some points to make about the innovativeness of the proposed research, please make them.

Training

This is where you tell the readers about you. How do you do this? You do it primarily in the training sections you write, in the research you propose, in the sections the sponsor(s)/mentor(s) write, in the letters of references, and in your biosketch. Let us start first with the training sections you write about yourself. They include:

- Goals for fellowship training and career (1 page maximum)
- Activities planned under the award (1 page maximum)
- Doctoral dissertation and other research experience (2 pages maximum)
- Respective contributions (1 page maximum)

TABLE 6.2 Primary Scored Criteria for Review of NIH NRSA Fellowship Applications

Overall Impact/Merit. Reviewers will provide an overall impact score to reflect their assessment of the likelihood that the fellowship will enhance the candidate's potential for, and commitment to, an independent scientific research career in a health-related field, in consideration of the scored and additional review criteria.

A fellowship application has a research project that is integrated with the training plan. The review will emphasize the applicant's potential for an independent, scientific research career, the applicant's need for the proposed training, and the degree to which the research project and training plan, the sponsor(s), and the environment will satisfy those needs.

Predoctoral NRSA (F31):

1. **Fellowship Applicant**
   Are the applicant's academic record and research experience of high quality? Does the applicant have the potential to develop into an independent and productive researcher in biomedical, behavioral, or clinical science? Does the applicant demonstrate commitment to a career as an independent researcher in the future?

2. **Sponsors, Collaborators, and Consultants**
   Are the sponsor(s') research qualifications (including recent publications) and track record of mentoring individuals at a similar stage appropriate for the needs of the applicant? Is there evidence of a match between the research interests of the applicant and the sponsor(s)? Do the sponsor(s) demonstrate an understanding of the applicant's training needs as well as the ability and commitment to assist in meeting these needs? Is there evidence of adequate research funds to support the applicant's proposed research project and training for the duration of the fellowship? If a team of sponsors is proposed, is the team structure well justified for the mentored training plan, and are the roles of the individual members appropriate and clearly defined? Are the qualifications of any collaborator(s) and/or consultant(s), including their complementary expertise and previous experience in fostering the training of fellows, appropriate for the proposed project?

3. **Research Training Plan**
   Is the proposed research plan of high scientific quality, and is it well integrated with the applicant's/proposed training plan? Is the research project consistent with the applicant's stage of research development? Is the proposed time frame feasible to accomplish the proposed research training? Based on the sponsor's description of his or her active research program, is the applicant's proposed research project sufficiently distinct from the sponsor's funded research for the applicant's career stage?

4. **Training Potential**
   Do the proposed research project and training plan have the potential to provide the applicant with the requisite individualized and mentored experiences that will develop his or her knowledge and research and professional development skills? Does the training plan take advantage of the applicant's strengths, and address gaps in needed skills? Does the training plan document a clear need for, and value of, the proposed training? Does the proposed research training have the potential to serve as a sound foundation that will facilitate the applicant's transition to the next career stage and enhance the applicant's ability to develop into an independent and productive research scientist?

5. **Institutional Environment and Commitment to Training**
   Are the research facilities, resources (e.g., equipment, laboratory space, computer time, subject populations), and training opportunities (e.g., seminars, workshops, professional development opportunities) adequate and appropriate? Is the institutional environment for the applicant's scientific development of high quality? Is there appropriate institutional commitment to fostering the applicant's mentored training toward his or her research career goals?

(continued)

TABLE 6.2 Primary Scored Criteria for Review of NIH NRSA Fellowship
Applications (*continued*)

Postdoctoral NRSA (F32):
Same, with the exception of No. 4:
  4. Training Potential
    Do the proposed research project and training plan have the potential to provide the
    applicant with the requisite individualized and mentored experiences that will develop
    his or her knowledge and research and professional development skills? Does the
    training plan take advantage of the applicant's strengths, and address gaps in needed
    skills? Does the training plan document a clear need for, and value of, the proposed
    training for the applicant? Does the proposed research training have the potential to
    serve as a sound foundation that will clearly lead the fellow to an independent and
    productive research career?

From the NIH (2010).

- Selection of sponsor and institution (1 page maximum)
- Training in the responsible conduct of research (1 page maximum)

What do you include in each section? First, be sure to look at the
Funding Opportunity Announcement (FOA) for the type of proposal
you wish to write. How do you find it? If you go to the main NIH
webpage (www.nih.gov), click on "Grants and Funding" and look in the
left-hand column, you will see "Types of Grant Programs." Click on it.
In the middle of the next page, you will see a box (scroll down if you do
not see it), which has as one option "Research Training and Fellowships
(T and F series)." Click on it. Then, under "Individual Fellowships" you
will see "F Kiosk." Click on it and you are there—at the bottom of the
page are links to the F31 and F32 FOAs! Read the one that is relevant for
you (predoctoral F31 or postdoctoral F32) and see what they ask you to
write in each section.

Look also at the SF424 (R&R) for fellowships—it too provides guidance about what you are to write. How do you find it? Go to the main NIH
webpage (www.nih.gov), click on "Grants and Funding," click on "Forms
and Applications" in the left-hand column, then click on SF424 (R&R).
Scroll down and you will see "Individual Fellowship Application Guide
SF424 (R&R)—Forms Version C." That is what you want! As of this writing,
the most recent version is dated 11/25/14. Be sure to examine the review
criteria for the grant you are interested in, because this will tell you what
reviewers are looking for (you can find a link to these in the F Kiosk mentioned earlier). Most helpful is reading examples of other recent successful
proposals—what did other folks include in each of the sections? Remember
that if you can improve upon what another person has done, do so—you
do not want to shoot for the lowest common denominator among those
who have been funded.

Goals for Fellowship Training and Career (1 Page Maximum)

The application guidelines say that in this section you should describe your overall career goals, explain how the proposed research training will enable you to attain these goals, and identify the skills, theories, conceptual approaches, and so on to be learned or enhanced during the award. You should have thought about your goals before writing the proposal, and you should be specific when writing about your goals. Talk about how you hope to contribute to research in your area. If you have planned a trajectory for your research, write about it—be clear, for example, that you are developing a program of research. If you plan to seek future funding, elaborate on this. If you are hoping to obtain a tenure-track academic position, say so. The goal is to convince reviewers that if they fund you, you will continue to contribute to research in your area.

Activities Planned Under the Award (1 Page Maximum)

The guidelines indicate that you should describe, by year, the activities (research, coursework, etc.) you will be involved in under the proposed award; estimate the percentage of time to be devoted to each activity; and describe activities other than research and relate them to the proposed training. From what you say in this section, along with what the sponsor(s)/mentor(s) say, reviewers will decide whether the training plan is related to the research plan, whether it is consistent with your stage of research development, and whether it will provide you with the individualized and supervised experiences to develop the research skills you need. They will also evaluate whether the proposed research training has the potential to serve as a sound foundation for a productive career. As mentioned earlier, be specific, but here it is about what you will learn and how you will learn it. Coursework is fine, but also include individualized work with your sponsor(s)/mentor(s) and other experts. Perhaps you will propose to be a research assistant (RA) on one of your mentor(s)' research projects; if so, exactly what will you do? And will you sit in regularly on one or more of your mentor's research team meetings so you can learn the ins and outs of doing research? If there are research institutes or centers close to you, will you participate in one or more that are relevant to your research? Perhaps you will propose to take courses, attend workshops, or participate in laboratory experiences to learn certain methods or analysis approaches. Consider attending research conferences, writing and/or making presentations, and co-authoring articles reporting research. Flesh out the activities of the training plan, but do not just say you will do *x*, *y*, and *z*; also say why you will do them—what you will learn and how they will help you with the research you will conduct now or in the future.

Although you only have a maximum of one page for this section, consider including two tables in your presentation: a table that summarizes your proposed training and indicates when each training activity will occur (Table 6.3) and a small table that shows the percentage of time you will spend on each major type of activity (Table 6.4). To save space, some people put their training goals in the text and organize the first table by those goals. Some people organize it by "time" (e.g., what they will do in each semester), and others organize it by type of activity (e.g., all coursework before individual activities). Some people include their research project in the timeline, while others choose not to. Others combine the two tables into one to save space. All of these approaches will work fine. However, (a) do not list things willy-nilly and expect reviewers to figure out what you are going to learn when, and what purpose it serves; and (b) be succinct so you can fit everything onto one page.

In addition, if you are writing a proposal for a predoctoral NRSA, our advice is that whatever you list in this section should go beyond what you will do for your traditional doctoral program; if you are just proposing to do what you would do anyway, why should NIH fund the fellowship? And as you become more senior (e.g., early predoctoral to more senior predoctoral to postdoctoral), you will have less formal coursework to take and more individualized activities and research to undertake. Thus, those later in their programs will want to emphasize research time instead of coursework listing time percentages. In addition, their research should be well developed because, with luck, they have learned most of the basics of designing good research in their coursework and early experiences.

Doctoral Dissertation and Other Research Experience *(2 Pages Maximum)*

In this section, you should summarize your research experiences in chronological order, including areas studied and conclusions reached; specify which were part of your thesis or dissertation. If you have no research experience, discuss other scientific experiences. Note that you do *not* list academic courses here. If you are early in your doctoral program, you should not (and will not be able to) include your doctoral dissertation here; if you are later in your doctoral program (i.e., you will have successfully completed comprehensive exams by the time of the award), you should include a narrative of the doctoral dissertation (although plans may be preliminary when you prepare the proposal). Reviewers will use the information you present here, in conjunction with the other information presented, to determine whether your research experience is of "high quality" and whether you have the potential to develop as an independent and productive researcher. So, have you been part of any studies? Were you an RA? Did you conduct studies as part of coursework? Have you participated in your mentor's research? Have

TABLE 6.3 Training Activities Planned During the Fellowship

Goal	Activity	Year 1 Fall	Year 1 Spr	Year 1 Sum	Year 2 Fall	Year 2 Spr	Year 2 Sum	Year 3 Fall	Year 3 Spr	Year 3 Sum
1. Gain knowledge about intervention design and analysis	Coursework: Nxxx: Title Byyy: Title	X	X							
	Shortcourse zzzzz			X						
	Participate in analysis of mentor's data				X	X	X			
	Participate in authoring presentations and articles on mentor's data						X	X	X	X
2. Gain knowledge about psychometrics	Coursework: Paaa: Title Pbbb: Title				X	X				
3. Gain competence in use of cortisol assessment	BBL workshop on cortisol assessment				X					
	Independent readings				X	X	X			
	Practice cortisol assessments; achieve reliability						X			
Etc.										

TABLE 6.4 Percentage of Time to Be Devoted to Each Major Activity During the Fellowship

Activity	Year 1	Year 2	Year 3
Research (%)	50	75	100
Coursework/Independent Study (%)	40	25	0
Teaching (TA) (%)	10	0	0
Clinical (%)	0	0	0
Total (%)	100	100	100

you been a principal investigator (PI) or co-investigator (Co-I) on any studies where you work? Were you a data collector? Subject recruiter? Site coordinator? For every experience, briefly say what the study was about; who the PI was; if funded, who funded it; what the main methods and findings were (if possible); what publications you were a part of (if relevant); and what your role was on the project—what you did and learned. What if you have not been part of any studies or not done any of these activities? You can then write about other scholarly work you have done related to the research topic. Perhaps you did an integrative literature review or a secondary analysis of existing data. Perhaps you have relevant clinical experience that informs your research (have you published any clinically focused articles?).

If the NRSA application is your first involvement in research, think carefully about your past and what you have done that might be relevant to the proposed research and training. Even if what you did was in a totally different topic area, if you learned something that is relevant for the research you hope to do, great—present it! Just be sure to identify what you learned and how it relates to the proposed NRSA.

You might want to write each piece of this section separately, then fit them together—or you might have written pieces in the past that you can crib from (it is fine to crib from yourself as long as it is not a published work). But watch out! The instructions say to present activities in chronological order, and that can be difficult if your research focus and interests have changed over the years. Do not just mash the pieces together; make sure they are in chronological order, then go back and make sure they all work together. And do not leave out work that might be in a different area—try to make it fit by saying what you learned from it.

Respective Contributions (1 Page Maximum)

This is the place where you describe the collaboration between you and your sponsor(s)/mentor(s) in the development, review, and editing of the research training plan—including the proposed research. You should also discuss the respective roles you will play in conducting the proposed research. Why in heaven's name would the NIH want to know about this? Because some pre- and postdoctoral individuals are hired labor on grants and the NIH does not want to support that kind of activity via an NRSA. They want this to be about *you*, your training, and your research. So your goal here is to note that you have done the work of writing the proposal (and it should be true!), but the sponsor(s)/mentor(s) were intimately involved—meeting with you, advising you, reading drafts, providing feedback, and so forth. Also, be clear that to accomplish the proposed research, you will do the work, but not alone. Your sponsor(s)/mentor(s) will meet with you regularly, advise you on the science and its management, help you resolve issues that arise, guide you in writing the dissertation or required report and subsequent publications, and so forth. Thus, they should play an active role in mentoring you throughout the project, but neither they nor anyone else should do the project for you. That is not to say that you cannot hire help or use help that is offered, but you should be in charge of your research project.

Selection of Sponsor and Institution (1 Page Maximum)

In this section, you describe the rationale for the selection of your sponsor and the institution at which you are studying. Explain why the sponsor/ mentor and co-sponsors/mentors, if any, were selected to accomplish the research training goals. Reviewers are interested in a number of things, but the most important is the *fit* between you and your sponsor(s)/mentor(s). Reviewers will also look closely at the sponsor(s)'/mentor(s)' qualifications to guide you: Are they established researchers in their areas—with funding and publications to support that determination? Are they a match to your research interests and needs? Do they have experience mentoring others? What opportunities can they provide to you? What about personal characteristics? (Are they supportive? Will they make themselves available when needed—can you get on their calendars?) There may be other things you would like to put in this section; if the points are relevant to what you are proposing, include them. However, do not create a sponsorship team based on just the school they are in or their availability; each person has to offer you something that you need in your proposed training and research. Ideally, the primary mentor will be in your school; if that person is not a content expert, perhaps you have selected her or him to mentor you in research methods or the development of a research career, writing for publication, or some other "generic" research topic. If so, make that clear.

The primary mentor may be an expert in the proposed content area, but your training goals may include learning about other areas (perhaps psychometrics, biobehavioral assessments, or intervention design) in which the primary mentor is not an expert. You will want the co-sponsors to have demonstrable expertise (via at least publications) in one or more of the areas you mention in your training plan. Make sure that collectively the sponsors/mentors meet the criteria noted earlier and that they have the expertise to guide your work. You might even want to include a more senior mentor to "mentor the mentors" who have not yet had the opportunity to mentor others. Remember, also, that not all of your mentors need to be at one institution; however, you do need to be clear about how you will work with mentors who are distant from you (travel? e-mail? Skype? a combination?), and in the Sponsor section, the mentors will have the opportunity to say how they will work together to guide you.

The institution should have been chosen because it allows you to study x, y, or z. If you are a predoctoral applicant, will the doctoral program and its coursework provide what you need to accomplish your goals? Does the school or university provide a research intensive setting? Will it provide you the opportunity to work with your sponsor(s)? Does it have research support services to help you with your research? Does the school or university have research institutes or centers in which you can become involved? The goal is to articulate the research strengths of the institution you have chosen. If your school does not have those strengths, perhaps another school within the institution will be able to provide them, or you can devise a training plan that includes travel to other institutions to work with noted experts. If the proposed research training is to take place at a site other than the sponsoring organization, provide an explanation here.

Let's be realistic. What if you chose the institution because it was near your home and the institution assigned you a mentor? That sort of thing usually would not fly in an NRSA application, so it is wise to think beyond these sorts of explanations. If you are not sure of your direction, you might want to use the early months of your predoctoral studies to determine where your interests lie and then seek out experts on your campus or nearby who can serve as mentors to you if there are none in your school. You might be able to take a course from these individuals and get to know them. If they are a good fit for your NRSA needs, you might want to show interest in their research, not only by asking questions but also by volunteering to work with them on selected studies. Also, are there relevant research institutes or centers on your campus or nearby? Might they provide a venue for getting to know senior researchers in your area through journal clubs, presentations, or meet-and-greet sessions? There are many ways to make these contacts, so do take advantage of them.

Responsible Conduct of Research (1 Page Maximum; Not Counted in 12-Page Total)

Responsible conduct of research (RCR) is defined as "the practice of scientific investigation with integrity" (NIH, 2009, Definition, para 1). It involves "the awareness and application of established professional norms and ethical principles in the performance of all activities related to scientific research" (NIH, 2009, Definition, para 1). Being "unaware" of professional norms is not an acceptable excuse—you must be aware of and apply appropriate ethics in conducting your research. NIH requires that every individual whom they support via fellowship or career development award (CDA) funding receive continued training in RCR. If you do not have a plan for obtaining training in RCR, your proposal may be delayed being reviewed or may not be reviewed at all.

Conducting research responsibly involves more than just treating human subjects well, although it includes that. It also includes knowing about conflict of interest issues; mentor–mentee responsibilities and relationships; collaborative research roles and responsibilities; peer review considerations; data acquisition, management, sharing, and ownership; research misconduct; responsible authorship; HIPAA (Health Insurance Portability and Accountability Act) rules; and so on. For example, did you know that the PI is responsible for the quality of the data collected by every person working on her or his study? What if the data records are not well protected and are hacked? What if an RA fabricates data? What if a subject has an adverse event? As the PI, will you be held responsible? You need to know, and this training should provide you with the information you need.

For those doing NIH fellowships and CDAs, a "notice" released in 2009 outlines what you are to include in this section of the proposal. It is NOT-OD-10-019, and you can find it on the NIH website. We encourage everyone who is considering applying for a fellowship to read it in detail (if the information is not in the FOA or the SF424 [R&R]) and include the requested information. You are asked to document prior participation or instruction in RCR (including the date each activity was completed), and propose plans to receive ongoing instruction in RCR—perhaps via something your sponsoring institution plans to provide, or through your own plans to obtain the content. The NIH also asks that the role of your sponsor(s)/mentor(s) in the instruction be described.

Instruction in RCR can occur both formally (through courses and seminars) and informally (e.g., face-to-face discussions or participation in research team meetings where data collection standards are assessed and discussed). The training should occur throughout the fellowship and cannot only be online or only be related to human subjects issues (e.g., via

Collaborative Institutional Training Initiative [CITI] training). In addition, the plans should be appropriate for your career stage. In the early stages of your fellowship, you will be a "learner," perhaps getting the content from courses you attend and small group discussions. As you become more senior, you will move from being "just" a learner to also being someone who teaches others. Indeed, if you are teaching research to any level of students, be sure to include it! Similarly, teaching RAs or other research personnel about appropriate conduct of research should be included.

The NIH requires you to address five foci for all of the RCR training you have taken in the past and will undertake during the award:

1. Format: Consider including coursework you will be taking (e.g., data analysis courses might cover data management issues; research courses might cover human subjects issues) as well as courses offered at your institution on RCR topics (perhaps the graduate school has such an offering); substantial face-to-face discussions with your sponsor(s)/ mentor(s) and among trainees; and participation of your sponsor(s)/ mentor(s) in this training.
2. Subject matter: Discussed earlier.
3. Faculty mentor participation: Describe how your mentor(s) contribute to formal and/or informal instruction of others and you.
4. Duration of instruction: The NIH specifies that fellows should have at least 8 contact hours during a fellowship, but we recommend that you consider describing at least some training across the entire grant period.
5. Frequency of instruction: Typically, reviewers will expect you to receive instruction (formally or informally) throughout the entire grant period.

You might want to make a table of what you have done and propose to do in each year of the award, crossed with these five foci.

When reviewers look at training in RCR, they rate it as either acceptable or unacceptable and do not factor their review of this section into your score. However, a proposal cannot be funded until the training plan is considered acceptable. So why not think it through and write it compellingly the first time? Then, once funded, *do what you propose*. This is not just an exercise in writing—it is a plan for you to always be on top of the current professional ethical standards.

Sponsor and Co-Sponsor Information

The sponsor(s) and co-sponsor(s) are collectively allowed up to six pages to cover five topics for each of them:

- Research Support Available
- Previous Fellows/Trainees

- Training Plan, Environment, Research Facilities
- Number of Fellows/Trainees to Be Supervised During the Fellowship
- Applicant's Qualifications and Potential for a Research Career

Research Support Available

In this section, sponsors should describe their current and pending research and research training support that will be available to you during the proposed training experience. Usually this information is put in a small table (for each sponsor) that identifies the source of the sponsor's support (funding source, identifying number, title, name of PI, and dates and amount of the award). For example, if one or more of your sponsors is a faculty member on a T32 (pre- and/or postdoctoral institutional training grant) that will provide training opportunities to you (e.g., a course, human subjects training) during the proposed award, it should be listed. If a sponsor is on or leading a research grant that will provide training opportunities for you (e.g., you may sit in on team meetings or perform secondary analysis of the data collected for the grant), the grants should be listed.

Previous Fellows/Trainees

Each sponsor and cosponsor should indicate the total number of predoctoral and postdoctoral individuals previously sponsored. Each should also select five sponsored individuals who are representative and provide their present employing organizations and position titles (or occupations). Ideally, you want to select folks who have sponsored lots of other NRSA fellows or T32 trainees, but what if that is not the case? The sponsors should be creative. Perhaps they have mentored young faculty researchers or predoctoral students or postdoctoral fellows who are not NRSA or T32 recipients. Rather than just saying that they have not sponsored any NRSA/T32 folks, they might add a statement about anyone else they have mentored.

Training Plan, Environment, and Research Facilities

The training plan about which the sponsor(s) write should go along with what you have written. If they are contradictory, the reviewers will know that you are not together on the plans and, therefore, you will not be funded; so make sure the two sections parallel one another. The instructions sound as if the sponsor(s) is (are) developing the plan for you, but our experience is that the sponsor(s) and applicant (you) usually develop the training plan together. Do not forget the types of things you have put in your training plan (e.g., classes, seminars, regular meetings with sponsor[s]' research teams, one-on-one time between sponsor[s] and you, laboratory experiences, RA experiences, opportunities for interaction with other groups and scientists). The sponsor(s) should be sure to describe the skills and techniques you will learn and indicate their relationship to your career goals.

In addition to the training you will undertake during the fellowship, the sponsor(s) should describe the research environment and research facilities and equipment that will be available to you. There is also a Facilities and Resources section required for the proposal, and some sponsor(s) choose to mimic that section here. Others use that section for more general institutional resources and use this section to describe what *they* will provide to your research training (perhaps they have a laboratory that will provide you with certain training or experiences or research equipment needed for your study, or they have data that they will make available to you).

Number of Fellows/Trainees to Be Supervised During the Fellowship

Sponsors and cosponsors are also asked to state the number of fellows and trainees they will supervise during your fellowship and indicate whether they are predoctoral students or postdoctoral fellows. Why in heaven's name would this matter? NIH does not want sponsors to be sponsoring too many people at once. If they are sponsoring a lot, there is a question about whether they will have time to mentor each of the individuals adequately.

Applicant's Qualifications and Potential for a Research Career

Lastly, the sponsor and cosponsors address your qualifications and potential for a research career. This is their reference for you (since they cannot be referees), and it is critical to your success. What they say must be strongly positive or you will not have a chance at getting the fellowship. For example, if the sponsor says you are mediocre or might someday make a competent researcher, this comment can be damning with faint praise and would not get you funded. Sponsors should enthusiastically describe how you are suited for this training opportunity based on your academic record and research experience. They should say how the research training plan and their own expertise will assist in making you an independent researcher.

We suggest that you ask your sponsors to write their sections early so you can read them. Critique and edit the sponsor(s)' sections just the way you do the rest of the proposal. Make sure that what the sponsors say and what you say in the training plan match. Sometimes sponsors may ask you to draft some sections for them; whether you agree to do so is up to you and your primary sponsor, but if, for example, you draft the section on your qualifications, this is not the time to be self-effacing and humble; however, do not just state that you are wonderful—show *how* you are wonderful based on your accomplishments and potential. We would also suggest that if you have more than one sponsor (and most people do), plans need to be included for how they will work together to mentor you. This is especially critical if one or more of the sponsors live and work at a distance from you and your primary sponsor.

As you can tell from the sections requested, reviewers will be trying to determine whether the sponsor(s) qualifications (including successful competition for research support) and track record of mentoring are appropriate for the proposed fellowship. They will want to know whether there is evidence of a match between your research interests and those of the sponsor(s), and whether the sponsor(s) have a demonstrated ability and commitment to meet your fellowship needs. They will determine whether the proposed research training has the potential to provide you with the individualized and supervised experiences needed to develop your research skills and provide you with a sound foundation for a productive research career. Of course, they will also want to make sure that the institution is committed to your research training and that research facilities, resources, and training opportunities are adequate and appropriate.

By the way, if you are applying for a predoctoral NRSA and your primary mentor and dissertation chair are different people, please add a support letter from the dissertation chair in the Other Attachments section. If you have an expert collaborating on the project or serving on your dissertation committee, you may also want a letter of support from that person. If someone will be providing access to a laboratory or other resource, consider adding a letter granting you such access. While these individuals do not participate in the various "sponsor" sections, their expertise and previous experience in training other fellows can be very helpful to you.

Additional Educational Information

For predoctoral fellowship applicants, the NIH now requires information about one's graduate program. In Other Attachments, the applicant's graduate program is to be described, including its structure, milestones and their timing, monitoring of student progress, and the average time to degree over the past 10 years. In addition to this general information, your progress in the program must be described. This information is typically provided by the graduate program director or the department chair, with the name of the individual providing the information included at the end of the presentation.

Letters of Reference

Letters of reference are typically not part of a research application (we are not talking about letters of support or consultant letters), but they are a required part of a fellowship application. They do not go *in* your grant application, but are submitted separately by the referee on your behalf. You are asked to get references from at least three, but no more than five, individuals who can speak knowledgeably about your qualifications, training, and interests. These cannot be individuals directly involved in the application (such as sponsors), who state their views in the sections described earlier.

The goal of these referees is to address your competence and potential to develop into an independent investigator. Therefore, select only folks who will (a) provide meaningful, relevant input; (b) be very, very positive; and (c) submit the reference on time (by the date the application is due to the NIH). They are asked to use up to two pages to address (a) your research ability and potential to become an independent researcher; (b) adequacy of your scientific background; (c) written and verbal communication abilities; (d) quality of your research endeavors or publications; (e) perseverance in pursing goals; (f) evidence of originality; (g) need for further research experience and training; and (h) familiarity with the research literature (NIH, 2014). Carefully select people who can address these topics.

You can help these people help you by asking them well in advance of the due date, giving them a copy of your biosketch or curriculum vitae (CV) so they are up to date on your accomplishments, and giving them at least an abstract of your proposed NRSA (preferably, you will be able to give them a copy of the Specific Aims for the research, your goals, and your training plan). You want them to speak knowledgeably not only about where you have been, but also about where you are going. Each referee is allowed two pages.

It is important that these letters are matched to the correct application, so you need to provide information about who these folks are in the cover letter to your application (include name, departmental affiliation, and institution) and to supply the referees with information on your electronic research administration commons (eRA Commons) user name, first and last names as they appear on your eRA Commons account, and the FOA number to which you are responding. Referees will submit their letters electronically through the eRA Commons, and the NIH will send confirmation emails to both the referees and to you so you know that the referees have submitted their evaluations.

SUMMARY

As you will notice when you read the guidelines for the SF424 (R&R) for fellowship applications and look at Table 6.1, there are many additional sections required for an NRSA, but we have covered the majority of them in this chapter and in the chapters on developing the rationale for your study and writing about the research design and methods (Approach). Do not forget, however, to read about Human Subjects, if you are going to have them, Biosketches, References, and so forth.

REFERENCES

National Institutes of Health (NIH). (2009, November). *Update on the requirement for instruction in the responsible conduct of research*. Retrieved from http://grants.nih.gov/grants/guide/notice-files/NOT-OD-10-019.html

National Institutes of Health (NIH). (2014, May). *Definitions of criteria and considerations for F critiques*. Retrieved from http://grants.nih.gov/grants/peer/critiques/f.htm

National Institutes of Health (NIH). (2014, November). *SF424 (R&R) Individual Fellowship Application Guide for NIH and AHRQ*. Retrieved from: http://grants.nih.gov/grants/funding/424/SF424_RR_Guide_Fellowship_VerC.pdf

SEVEN

CAREER DEVELOPMENT AWARD PROPOSALS

Many different agencies offer career development awards (CDAs)—for development as a researcher, either bench or bedside, in a particular topic area or not; for development as a faculty member or as a practitioner; and so on. CDAs are usually reserved for folks early in their careers who wish (and need) to obtain additional training as well as to do a project that is foundational for their continued success, or for those who wish to switch their topic area to a new one. Applications usually require you to expound not solely on the project to be conducted, but also on yourself because the purpose of the award is to fund you to become an independent investigator, practitioner, teacher, and so on. *You* are as important as the project you propose, as is your *need* for the award. These awards come in all shapes and sizes (e.g., from the National Institutes of Health [NIH; K awards], the American Cancer Society [ACS], and the Robert Wood Johnson [RWJ] Foundation), and you are encouraged to read the guidelines very carefully for the award you are interested in, to be sure you cover everything the funder wishes. It is also wise to read the review criteria so you do not leave anything out.

NATIONAL INSTITUTES OF HEALTH

The NIH has a number of career development opportunities for those interested in health-related research. These usually have an activity designation that begins with a "K," and to learn more about these opportunities, you are encouraged to visit the K kiosk at the NIH website (www.nih.gov; use the "search" function to find whatever you wish, such as the K kiosk). On the K-kiosk page, under Career Award Policy Issues in the Policies and Notices section, you will find the Career Award Wizard, which can be quite helpful as you decide which, if any, of the K awards might be right for you. It also has transcripts of podcasts, Funding Opportunity Announcements (FOAs), and other helpful information. Read carefully, because not all institutes at the NIH participate in all of the possible K awards, cover the same number of years of funding, or offer the same level of financial support. For example, the National Institute of Nursing Research (NINR), which is one of the NIH's institutes, participates only in the K01, K23, K24, and K99/R00 awards at this time. (The NINR has a great table of its funding mechanisms, which can be found on its website at www.ninr.nih.gov in the Office of Extramural Programs section.) You are also encouraged to contact a scientific program officer at the institutes in which you are interested; these people have a wealth of knowledge and can be most helpful when you are trying to navigate the NIH offerings.

The K01 is a general mentored research scientist development award, while the K23, also a mentored award, is designed for those whose research is patient oriented. The K99/R00, or Pathway to Independence Award, is for those who are postdoctoral candidates or in nontenure-track faculty positions and wish a mentored period followed by an independent period of research support. The K24 is for those who are midcareer (associate professor or equivalent), actively funded to do patient-oriented research, and wish to mentor others with the K award. You should read about each of these opportunities in the FOA section of the K kiosk. All of the K awards use the SF424 (R&R) application format, which can also be found on the NIH website. Be sure to read the general SF424 (R&R) instructions as well as the section that has supplemental instructions specifically for those applying for CDA/K awards.

The K01 and K23 are designed for individuals who have already earned the terminal degree in their field and need support for two reasons: (a) to obtain additional training in order to design and conduct the research in which they are interested, and (b) to be able to conduct a preliminary or small research project to get the next phase of their research off the ground. If you do not need further training or if you are ready to move on to a research project, you are probably *not* a good fit for a CDA—you might be ready to move straight to research funding.

Note that some of the K awards are "mentored" awards—meaning that you are not in this alone. You need to identify strong mentors who can (and will) provide you with the training you need to have a successful career. As you will see, these mentors are a very important part of the application. In addition, a CDA requires substantial commitment on the part of the institution where you propose doing the award. Therefore, the NIH is typically interested in situations where the institution has a commitment to continuing to employ the candidate for some time to come. How does this translate into typical academic-ese? Usually, applicants will be individuals who have been accepted to or already are on the tenure track. If you are in a nontenurable position in a clinical agency or educational institution, you might want to contact an NIH program officer to discuss your situation before you spend the time working on a proposal (and do read the K99/R00 FOA to see if that is a fit for your situation).

Typically, it is not reasonable to indicate that you will be offered a tenure-track slot *if* you get the CDA. The CDA is designed for those who already have such a commitment from an institution—not as a negotiating tool.

NIH requires that the individual applying for the award agree to commit 75% of her or his time to the award, year round, for 3 to 5 years. Since "year round" means for 12 months of the year, 75% of 12 months equals 9 months of commitment. You will need to commit 75% of your time to the award during the academic year and during the summer as well. Look carefully at the FOA to be sure that the money being offered will indeed cover 75% of your time. If it will not, you will need a contribution from your institution to cover the difference. Be sure to get this commitment in advance, before you do all the work of preparing an application.

As noted, there are both training and research components to the award, so in the application, you will write about each of these (see Table 7.1 for an overview of the main sections you will write, and Table 7.2 for the criteria reviewers will have in mind as they read these proposals). With the exception of a few notes, given in the following, you will follow the research sections of this book for the research sections of the proposal. We focus here on the additional sections the NIH desires for K applications. First is the information about you.

CANDIDATE INFORMATION

For the NIH, you are called "the candidate," and the information requested about you includes your (the candidate's):

1. Background
2. Career Goals and Objectives
3. Plan for Career Development/Training Activities During the Award Period
4. Training in the Responsible Conduct of Research

Let us discuss each of these in turn.

Background

It is important to remember that the NIH early-career CDAs are designed to support your becoming an independent investigator; you are not trying

TABLE 7.1 Selected Components of National Institutes of Health
Career Development Award Proposals

Title (200 characters and spaces maximum)

Summary
   a. Abstract (1 page; we recommend 30 lines)
   b. Project Narrative (2 to 3 sentences)

Introduction
   1. Introduction to Application (Resubmission Applications Only) (1 page maximum)

Candidate Information (12 pages maximum for Nos. 2 to 4 and 12)
   2. Candidate's Background
   3. Career Goals and Objectives
   4. Candidate's Plan for Career Development/Training Activities During Award Period
   5. Training in the Responsible Conduct of Research (1 page maximum)
   6. Candidates Plan to Provide Mentoring (only if required by FOA, thus only for select Ks) (6 pages maximum)

Statements and Letters of Support
   7. Plans and Statements of Mentor and Co-mentor(s) (6 pages maximum)
   8. Letters of Support from Collaborators, Contributors, and Consultants (6 pages maximum)

Environment and Institutional Commitment to Candidate
   9. Description of Institutional Environment (1 page maximum)
   10. Institutional Commitment to Candidate's Research Career Development (1 page maximum)

Research Plan
   11. Specific Aims (1 page maximum)
   12. Research Strategy (12 pages maximum for Candidate sections 2–4 and Research section 12 [Research Strategy])
       a. Significance
       b. Innovation
       c. Approach
          (Include Preliminary Studies where most appropriate)

Progress Report Publication List (for Renewal Applications Only)

Human Subjects Sections
   14. Protection of Human Subjects
   15. Inclusion of Women and Minorities (Planned Enrollment Report)
   16. Inclusion of Children

Other Research Plan Sections
   17. Vertebrate Animals
   18. Select Agent Research
   19. Consortium/Contractual Arrangements
   20. Resource Sharing Plan (sometimes)

Other
   21. Appendix

(continued)

TABLE 7.1 Selected Components of National Institutes of Health
Career Development Award Proposals *(continued)*

Biosketches
    a. Candidate (You)
    b. Mentor(s), Co-mentor(s), Other Senior/Key Persons

Budget
    c. SF424 R&R budget (only a few categories are used)
    d. Budget Justification

Etc.
Bibliography and References Cited
Facilities & Other Resources
Equipment
List of Referees
Letters of Reference (3–5, submitted separately)

Note: Content has been reorganized a bit and not all components are listed—just the major ones from the SF424 (R&R); the FOA always takes precedence. FOA, Funding Opportunity Announcement.

to make the case that you already know everything and do not need the CDA. The NIH is interested in your background as it relates to the research you propose doing now and in the future. They do not particularly care that you trained your pet hamster when you were a child unless it is relevant to the proposed research, so focus on what you have done that is relevant to your planned program of research. (Note: There is no particular page length for the Background section, but the Background, Career Goals and Objectives, and Career Development/Training During the Award all count toward the 12 pages that also include your research plan [Specific Aims are separate, as is Training in the Responsible Conduct of Research].)

While the NIH guidelines indicate that you should just include information that is not on the biosketch, and reviewers will read this section along with the biosketch, you want to tell a coherent story about your background, and jumping around to avoid things listed on the biosketch might make this section difficult to read. Be sure to (a) show that you are committed to a health-related research career; (b) describe your prior training and how it relates to your objectives for the CDA and your long-term career plans; (c) fold in your clinical focus, expertise, and background when they are a fit to the proposed topic; (d) show evidence of your ability to interact and collaborate with others; and (e) show your potential to develop into an independent, lead investigator. What sorts of things are we talking about? Well, let us say you have had lots of clinical experience in the neonatal intensive care unit (NICU) and your proposed goals relate to premature infants—tie these together so that your experience helps make the case for your strength in this area. Perhaps you have worked with elderly folks in a nursing home and you are now proposing a career as a tenure-track faculty member focused on gerontology—you might wish to show how your earlier experiences led

TABLE 7.2 Primary Scored Criteria for Review of the National Institutes of Health
Career Development Award Proposals

Overall Impact. Reviewers should provide their assessment of the likelihood that the
proposed career development and research plan will enhance the candidate's potential for
a productive, independent scientific research career in a health-related field, taking into
consideration the following criteria in determining the overall impact score.

Mentored Research Scientist Development Award (K01)

1. Candidate
  - Does the candidate have the potential to develop as an independent and productive
    researcher?
  - Are the candidate's prior training and research experience appropriate for this
    award?
  - Is the candidate's academic, clinical (if relevant), and research record of high quality?
  - Is there evidence of the candidate's commitment to meeting the program objectives to
    become an independent investigator in research?
  - Do the letters of reference address the preceding review criteria, and do they provide
    evidence that the candidate has a high potential for becoming an independent
    investigator?

2. Career Development Plan/Career Goals and Objectives/Plan to Provide Mentoring
  - What is the likelihood that the plan will contribute substantially to the scientific
    development of the candidate and lead to scientific independence?
  - Are the content, scope, phasing, and duration of the career development plan
    appropriate when considered in the context of prior training/research experience and
    the stated training and research objectives for achieving research independence?
  - Are there adequate plans for monitoring and evaluating the candidate's research and
    career development progress?

3. Research Plan
  - Are the proposed research question, design, and methodology of significant scientific
    and technical merit?
  - Is the research plan relevant to the candidate's research career objectives?
  - Is the research plan appropriate to the candidate's stage of research development and as
    a vehicle for developing the research skills described in the career development plan?

4. Mentor(s), Co-mentor(s), Consultant(s), Collaborator(s)
  - Are the qualifications of the mentor(s) in the area of the proposed research appropriate?
  - Does the mentor(s) adequately address the candidate's potential and his or her
    strengths and areas needing improvement?
  - Is there adequate description of the quality and extent of the mentor's proposed role in
    providing guidance and advice to the candidate?
  - Is the mentor's description of the elements of the research career development
    activities, including formal course work, adequate?
  - Is there evidence of the mentor's, consultant's, and/or collaborator's previous
    experience in fostering the development of independent investigators?
  - Is there evidence of the mentor's current research productivity and peer-reviewed support?
  - Is active/pending support for the proposed research project appropriate and adequate?
  - Are there adequate plans for monitoring and evaluating the career development
    awardee's progress toward independence?

(continued)

TABLE 7.2 Primary Scored Criteria for Review of the National Institutes of Health
Career Development Award Proposals *(continued)*

5. Environment and Institutional Commitment to the Candidate

- Is there clear commitment of the sponsoring institution to ensure that a minimum of 9 person-months (75% of the candidate's full-time professional effort) will be devoted directly to the research and career development activities described in the application, with the remaining percent effort being devoted to an appropriate balance of research, teaching, administrative, and clinical responsibilities?
- Is the institutional commitment to the career development of the candidate appropriately strong?
- Are the research facilities, resources, and training opportunities, including faculty capable of productive collaboration with the candidate, adequate and appropriate?
- Is the environment for scientific and professional development of the candidate of high quality?
- Is there assurance that the institution intends the candidate to be an integral part of its research program as an independent investigator?

Mentored Patient-Oriented Research Career Development Award (K23)

1. Candidate

- Does the candidate have the potential to develop as an independent and productive researcher?
- Are the candidate's prior training and research experience appropriate for this award?
- Is the candidate's academic, clinical (if relevant), and research record of high quality?
- Is there evidence of the candidate's commitment to meeting the program objectives to become an independent investigator in patient-oriented research?
- Do the letters of reference address the preceding review criteria, and do they provide evidence that the candidate has a high potential for becoming an independent investigator?

2. Career Development Plan/Career Goals and Objectives/Plan to Provide Mentoring

- What is the likelihood that the plan will contribute substantially to the scientific development of the candidate and lead to scientific independence?
- Are the content, scope, phasing, and duration of the career development plan appropriate when considered in the context of prior training/research experience and the stated training and research objectives for achieving research independence?
- Are there adequate plans for evaluating the candidate's research and career development progress?

3. Research Plan

- Are the proposed research question, design, and methodology of significant scientific and technical merit?
- Is the research plan relevant to the candidate's research career objectives?
- Is the research plan appropriate to the candidate's stage of research development and as a vehicle for developing the research skills described in the career development plan?

4. Mentor(s), Co-mentor(s), Consultant(s), Collaborator(s)

- Are the mentor's research qualifications in the area of the proposed research appropriate?
- Do(es) the mentor(s) adequately address the candidate's potential and his or her strengths and areas needing improvement? Is there adequate description of the quality and extent of the mentor's proposed role in providing guidance and advice to the candidate?

(continued)

TABLE 7.2 Primary Scored Criteria for Review of the National Institutes of Health
Career Development Award Proposals *(continued)*

- Is there adequate description of the quality and extent of the mentor's proposed role in providing guidance and advice to the candidate? Is the mentor's description of the elements of the research career development activities, including formal course work, adequate?
- Is there evidence of the mentor's, consultant's, and/or collaborator's previous experience in fostering the development of independent investigators?
- Is there evidence of the mentor's current research productivity and peer-reviewed support?
- Is active/pending support for the proposed research project appropriate and adequate?
- Are there adequate plans for monitoring and evaluating the career development awardee's progress toward independence?

5. **Environment and Institutional Commitment to the Candidate**
   - Is there clear commitment of the sponsoring institution to ensure that the required minimum of the candidate's effort will be devoted directly to the research described in the application, with the remaining percent effort being devoted to an appropriate balance of research, teaching, administrative, and clinical responsibilities?
   - Is the institutional commitment to the career development of the candidate appropriately strong?
   - Are the research facilities, resources, and training opportunities, including faculty capable of productive collaboration with the candidate, adequate and appropriate?
   - Is the environment for scientific and professional development of the candidate of high quality?
   - Is there assurance that the institution intends the candidate to be an integral part of its research program as an independent investigator?

From the NIH (2010).

to your interest in pursuing gerontological research topics. Even personal experiences might have led to your research interests. Your prior training might include stints as a research assistant; perhaps you completed a paper in a course that was relevant to the proposed CDA, or maybe you have been part of a working group that focuses on research topics related to your CDA. Did you co-author presentations or publications reporting results of research? Did you recruit participants for someone else's study or present research results to communities of participants? Each of these may be valuable in showing that you have been actively involved in research, that you collaborated successfully with others, and that you completed the work and reported it to the interested community. As a beginning researcher, no one is expecting your research assistantship to include the duties that a lead investigator would have, but perhaps you learned important skills about data collection, organizing instruments, entering data or something similar. The goal is to report activities from which you gained relevant skills, not to say that you already know everything. You want to show a sustained interest and growth over time (including presenting and publishing), but also show that you *need* the CDA to become an independent investigator.

Career Goals and Objectives

As noted earlier, the purpose of a CDA is to help you become an independent investigator in an important area. Therefore, do not just make a generic statement such as "my goal is to become an independent, funded investigator." Be specific about your topic and what you will do to further the science during your years as an independent investigator after the CDA. Perhaps the CDA is designed to help you learn how to develop and evaluate interventions to improve medication adherence in patients with diabetes, and the research is a preliminary study of an intervention you will further develop during the CDA. If so, build on that topic by writing that you will take what you learn and the results from the preliminary study done during the CDA to refine the intervention and conduct a full clinical trial of its efficacy (perhaps via subsequent research funding). Show a logical progression from your prior training to what will occur during the award, to your future goals/objectives as an independent researcher. You want to justify the need for further training in order to meet your goals/ objectives.

While the NIH says to include "past scientific history" in this section, if you have already covered it all in the Background section, details are not needed here—there usually is not room for repetition. The NIH also asks you to indicate how the award fits into past and future research career development, whether there are consistent themes or issues in your work, and, if your work has changed direction, to specify the reasons for the change. Most importantly, justify the award—explain how it will enable you to develop or expand your research career. Lastly, a timeline from the past through the CDA and subsequent grant support is helpful.

Candidate's Plan for Career Development/Training Activities During the Award Period

Now we get to the training you are proposing to undertake during the CDA. This section will overlap with what your mentors write, but that is okay. However, the two sections should *not* contradict one another—they need to be consistent in what they say your training will be and how it will occur during the award. Remember that you are not a student—you are proposing the CDA while you will be a tenure-track faculty member. So, unlike fellowship training plans, the training plan for a CDA will focus more on mentored-learning experiences than on formal courses (not that you might not have some of the latter—it is just that there will probably be fewer than when you were a doctoral student or fellow).

In what areas do you need training? Only you and your mentors can say and write a proposal that wraps the training and the research together. However, folks in the past have been funded for everything from learning how to design and evaluate interventions, to learning instrument development and psychometrics; developing or learning to use electronic mechanisms to intervene or assess relevant dimensions or perhaps learning about cost–benefit analysis approaches; learning a new language or culture or perhaps learning advanced analytic techniques; learning a new methodological approach or learning a relevant field (e.g., genetics). It is important that (a) what you propose to learn is important to the research you hope to conduct, and (b) you have not had such training in the past. It is not wise to say that you want to learn, for example, advanced analytic techniques that you have already had in class but just did not learn or pay attention to. This is not "makeup work"—it is an opportunity to enhance your ability to conduct cutting-edge research and expand your scientific horizons. In the text, you need to explain how each training activity is related to your proposed research and career development plans.

In this section of the proposal, talk about *how* you will go about learning what is important. Emphasize the new and enhanced research skills and knowledge you will acquire. Do include structured activities such as courses, but at this level your training should move beyond traditional coursework. You might want to include independent studies; regular meetings with your mentor(s) that include one-on-one discussions of research design, methods, analyses, human subjects issues, and so forth; if your mentor(s) are actively doing research, you might want to talk about becoming part of their research team(s) and participating in regular team meetings; developing presentations and articles from your study and/or co-presenting or co-authoring from your participation in your mentor(s)' research; attending conferences; analyzing existing data; and so forth. Consider summarizing all of your training activities in a table to accompany the text so the reviewers can see at a glance what you will be doing. First, organize your activities by content area so that it makes sense to the reviewers. Table 7.3 provides an example of a table you can personalize.

Lastly, the NIH asks that you specify the percentage of time you will spend on each type of activity each year of the award and explain how the activity is related to the proposed development plan and research. Your goal is to show a pattern of activity that moves from more heavily "training" activities to more heavily "research" activities across the award period. For example, you might have a table (along with explanatory text) that looks something like Table 7.4.

Your table might be quite different from this. Instead of teaching, or in addition to it, you might have a clinical or administrative role to fulfill. Whatever you will be doing, chart it and in the text explain how it will relate to your research training. For example, maybe you will have a clinical role in the pediatric intensive care unit (ICU) or teach a pediatric course, and your proposed CDA is to learn how to develop an intervention for children to better manage their chronic illnesses. Tie your anticipated work to the CDA.

TABLE 7.3 Sample Table of Training Activities Planned During the Career Development Award

Activity	Year 1			Year 2			Year 3		
	Fall	Spr	Sum	Fall	Spr	Sum	Fall	Spr	Sum
Longitudinal Methods and Analysis									
Course: Bxxx—Longitudinal Methods	X								
Course: Nxxx—Application of Longitudinal Approaches		X							
Collaborate on Mentor's Existing Longitudinal Project									
Participate in weekly team meetings	X	X	X						
Conduct analyses		X	X						
Co-author and make presentations				X	X	X	X		
Co-author Articles				X	X	X	X		
Measuring Allostatic Load									
Laboratory experience				X					
Independent study with xxx					X	X			
Practice assessments						X			
Etc.									

TABLE 7.4 Sample Table of Percentage of Time to Be Devoted to Each Major Activity During the Award

Activity	Year 1	Year 2	Year 3
Training (%)	50	30	10
Research (%)	25	45	65
Teaching (%)	25	25	25
Clinical (%)	0	0	0
Total (%)	100	100	100

Training in the Responsible Conduct of Research

The responsible conduct of research (RCR) is defined as "the practice of scientific investigation with integrity" and it involves "the awareness and application of established professional norms and ethical principles in the performance of all activities related to scientific research" (NIH, 2009, Definition, para 1). Thus, do not claim to be unaware of the professional norms in your field, because this is not an acceptable excuse. The NIH requires that every individual whom it supports via fellowship or CDA funding receives continued training in the responsible conduct of research.

Conducting research responsibly involves treating human subjects well, but it also includes knowing about the broader issues of conducting research ethically—maintaining rigor in the process of conducting the study, data collection standards, following the Health Insurance Portability and Accountability Act (HIPAA) rules, handling research misconduct of one's staff, rules of responsible authorship, and so forth. What are your responsibilities if you are the principal investigator (PI) of a project? Are you responsible for the quality of the intervention provided by your interveners? For the quality of the data collected by your research assistants (RAs)? What if a subject has an adverse event? Will you, as the PI, be held responsible? You need to know all of these things and many more; the ongoing training you outline should be designed to provide you with the information you need.

The NIH released a "notice" in 2009 that outlines what you are to include in this section of the proposal. It is NOT-OD-10-019 and is available on the NIH website (just click on the Grants and Funding link and enter the full NOT number in the box provided for NIH Grants and Contracts). We would encourage everyone who is considering applying for a CDA to read the notice in detail and be sure to include the requested information. (Key information is also covered in each relevant FOA the NIH announces.)

Instruction in RCR can occur both formally (through things such as courses and seminars) and informally (e.g., face-to-face discussions or participation in research team meetings where data collection standards are discussed and assessed). The training should occur throughout the CDA and cannot only be online or only be related to human subjects issues (e.g., via Collaborative Institutional Training Initiative [CITI] training). In addition, the plans should be appropriate for the applicant's stage of development. As you become more senior, you will move from being "just" a learner also to being someone who teaches others. Indeed, if you are teaching research to any level of student, be sure to include it. Similarly, teaching RAs or other research personnel about appropriate conduct of research should also be included.

The NIH requires you to address five foci for all of the RCR training you have taken in the past and will undertake during the award:

1. Format: At the CDA level, you will probably want to describe face-to-face discussions, didactic and small-group discussions, and independent study as well as any formal course work you will undertake that covers RCR topics.
2. Subject matter: Consider all aspects of RCR (e.g., conflict of interest, achieving and maintaining research standards and data quality, protection of human subjects); see NOT-OD-10-019 for a list of topics to consider.
3. Faculty mentor participation: It is important that your mentor(s) participate in teaching others (and you) about conducting research responsibly; describe that participation here.
4. Duration of instruction: The NIH does not specify a particular duration of RCR training for the CDAs, but consider describing at least some training across the entire grant period.
5. Frequency of instruction: The NIH also does not specify a particular frequency of RCR training for the CDAs, but we would recommend that you plan to receive or give instruction (formally or informally) each semester of the grant.

You might want to make a table of what you have done and propose to do each year of the award crossed with these five foci.

While reviewers rate your section on Training in the Responsible Conduct of Research as either acceptable or unacceptable and do not factor their review of this section into your score, the NIH has decided that (a) if you do not include this section, your proposal will not be reviewed, and (b) even if you do include it, if it is found to be inadequate, your proposal will not be funded until the plan is considered acceptable. So why not think it through and write it compellingly the first time? Once funded *do what you propose*. This is not just an exercise in writing—it is a plan for you always to be on top of current professional ethical standards. In addition, you will be asked to report annually on what you have done in this area.

Statements and Letters of Support

Plans and Statements of Mentor and Co-Mentor(s)

These statements are written by your primary mentor and co-mentors, if you have them. They are allowed a total of six pages to say how they will contribute to your (the candidate's) development. Included are (a) plans for your training and research career development, which should include the research to be conducted as well as other developmental activities such as seminars, scientific meetings, presentations, publications, training in the responsible conduct of research, and what you will be "allowed" to take when it is over (if, e.g., you propose working exclusively on mentors' research projects, the data may not be yours to take); (b) sources of support for the candidate, which are particularly important if the K budget will not cover everything that is needed on the project (e.g., will the mentor be providing a necessary laboratory in which you will conduct your research or equipment that will allow you to do your research?); (c) the nature and extent of supervision, which shows the commitment of mentors to the candidate's development; (d) the candidate's responsibilities during the award period—including research time, teaching load, clinical assignments, and service duties (e.g., committee work and administrative roles); and (e) plans for transitioning the candidate to independence (so you won't be a "trainee" forever).

It is important that this section identifies all mentors for the CDA. Each person's role in what is proposed and each person's anticipated contributions should be specified. If there are co-mentors, it is important that they indicate what their respective areas of expertise are, how they will share responsibility for the candidate's career development with the primary mentor, and how the mentors will work together. Resources that the co-mentors will commit to the CDA should also be described.

What the mentors say in this section should mesh seamlessly with what you (the candidate) say in the career development/training section. If there is a mismatch, reviewers will begin to wonder whether you are on the same page. The mentors should also use this opportunity to describe their previous mentoring experiences, including the type of mentoring, the number of persons they have mentored, and the career outcomes of those individuals. (Clearly, you should be productive with this award and thereafter, since your career successes will evaluated as part of the applications of future mentees.)

When preparing any section of an application, it is important to examine not just what information is requested but also what reviewers will expect in the section. For example, the reviewers for K awards are asked to indicate whether the mentor(s) have adequately addressed the candidate's potential, strengths, and areas needing improvement. Reviewers are also asked to address whether there are adequate plans to monitor and evaluate the candidate's progress toward independence. Thus, mentor(s) should be sure to address these topics in their statement(s) of support. If mentor(s) feel that the CDA applicant is not a strong candidate, the proposal will probably not do well in review.

Some folks choose to provide the information in this section in a joint statement from all of the mentors. Others choose to have each mentor write a letter to be included in the section; whatever you do, do not go over the six-page limit for the primary mentor and all co-mentors. If individual letters are used, each person will sign his or her own letter; if a joint statement is used, it might be wise to have all of the mentors sign the joint statement so it is clear that they agree with it.

It is important to think carefully when you are selecting your mentor(s). You want individuals who, first and foremost, are a fit with your training/research needs. But they should also be successful in obtaining extramural funding for their research and be currently funded if at all possible, publish what they find, provide appropriate training opportunities, work well together, and follow through with what they say they will do. You will not be happy if you have "wedded" yourself to a mentor who does not have time for you or does not follow through in training you. (Together, you should stick doggedly to your timeline once you get the award.) You do not necessarily need to find all the expertise and skills in one person—you can develop a team of mentors who collaborate to provide the variety of training you need. And you do not need to find all of these individuals in your school or institution. You can be creative in assembling a mentorship team that collectively have the expertise you need, but be sure to describe how you will work with each person and how the mentors will come together (electronically? at conferences?) to appropriately mentor and evaluate you.

Letters of Support From Collaborators, Contributors, and Consultants

In addition to your mentorship team, you may plan to have others involved in your training or research. Perhaps you will have consultants who will be less involved than the mentors but have important expertise to offer the proposed project. Perhaps a biostatistician or psychometrician will play a key role in your study, or perhaps you will have a substantive collaborator or two. While these individuals may not be identified as mentors and, thus are not part of the six-page mentors' statement already discussed, they have an opportunity to contribute to the application through letters of support that you add to the application. A total of six pages are allowed for all of these letters. The individuals who write them should describe how they will contribute to the project and their willingness to do so. If a fee is to be charged, that should be described as well. We would recommend that you consider asking these folks to write at least a bit about your strengths and what a wonderful research career you have in front of you.

Environment and Institutional Commitment

Description of Institutional Environment

This is a bit tricky because it may feel as if this section overlaps with another section of the proposal (Facilities and Other Resources). And indeed, the sections may overlap, but the NIH suggests that you refer to what is discussed in Facilities and Other Resources and say here how those facilities will be made available to the applicant. You should also describe research programs at the institution that are related to your area(s) of interest, and even list the faculty involved in these programs. Will there be chances for intellectual interactions with these individuals? If so, describe them here. For example, your institution may have research centers where everyone who is interested in a certain topic comes together for quarterly presentations, monthly article discussion sessions, informal interactions, and so forth. Describe all of these in this section. (One page is allowed for this section.)

Institutional Commitment to Candidate's Career Development

The institution has one page to document (in detail) its commitment to your development. This is usually in the form of a letter that is signed by your dean or chairperson (we would recommend that the two individuals cosign the letter). You want these people to say that you are a strong candidate for the CDA, indicate their wholehearted support of your application, agree to provide you with the requested release time, and describe the other duties they will ask of you during the award period. They should discuss *how* they will provide you with the necessary release time (e.g., will they be hiring someone else to take some of your teaching duties?). They should also make it clear that the school/institution is providing you the necessary office, laboratories, research space, computer access, and other resources that you need for the training and research. If appropriate, these individuals should provide you access to the population(s) you will study. (If it is not appropriate for them to grant this right, you will want support letters from the clinical sites granting such access.) Also, since the mentor(s) of your application will not be paid by the NIH to mentor you, agreement to provide the mentors time to mentor you is needed. If the mentors are in your department, the chairperson and dean can indicate that they will support the mentor in this endeavor. If some of your mentors are from other departments or schools, you may want their chairpersons to sign this letter as well.

Research

The research project you propose in a CDA is usually fairly preliminary in nature, allowing you to apply your training to the research project. You may even be working with secondary data or on a mentor's project in order to acquire skills and lay the foundation for research you will conduct after the CDA. Chapter 5 of this book will help you address the research component of a CDA.

Letters of Reference

Letters of reference are typically not part of a research application (we are not talking about letters of support or consultant letters), but they are a required part of a CDA application. They do not go *in* your grant, but are submitted separately by the referee on your behalf. You are asked to get references from at least three, but no more than five, individuals who can speak knowledgeably about your qualifications, training, and interests. These cannot be individuals directly involved in the application (such as mentors), because these individuals have a chance to state their views in the sections described earlier.

The goal of these referees is to address your competence and potential to develop into an independent investigator. Therefore, select only people who will (a) provide meaningful, relevant input; (b) be *very, very* positive; and (c) submit the reference on time (which is by the date the application is due to the NIH). They are asked to address (a) your potential for becoming an independent researcher; (b) evidence of your originality; (c) adequacy of your scientific background; (d) the quality of your research endeavors and/or publications; (e) your commitment to a health-oriented career; and (f) your need for further training and research experience. Therefore, carefully select people who can address these topics (in addition to any other comments they would like to make; NIH, 2014).

You can help these people help you by asking them well in advance of the due date, giving them a copy of your biosketch or curriculum vita (CV) so they are up to date on your accomplishments, and giving them at least an abstract of your proposed CDA (preferably, you will be able to give them a copy of the Specific Aims for the research, your goals, and your training plan). You want them to speak knowledgeably not only about where you have been, but also about where you are going. When possible, these individuals should be outside your current department. Each referee is allowed two pages.

It is important that these letters get matched to the correct application, so you are asked to provide information about who these folks are in your application (including name, departmental affiliation, and institution) and to supply the referees with information (including your electronic research administration commons [eRA Commons] user name, first and last names as they appear on your eRA Commons account, and the FOA number to which you are responding). Referees will submit their letters electronically through the eRA Commons, and the NIH will send confirmation emails to both the referees and to you so you know that the referees have submitted their evaluations of you.

OTHER NIH K AWARDS

As mentioned earlier, the NIH's CDAs come in many shapes and sizes. Explore all that are relevant for you and speak with the program officers at the institutes in which you are interested. However, we would like to mention the K12 (and KL2) programs. In these cases, the NIH makes awards to institutions so that they, in turn, can make the CDAs to individuals. Each institution has its own application form, but typically they request information similar to what we have covered here, and typically they are for mentored research and training experiences.

REFERENCES

National Institutes of Health (NIH). (2009, November). *Update on the requirement for instruction in the responsible conduct of research.* Retrieved from http://grants.nih.gov/grants/guide/notice-files/NOT-OD-10-019.html

National Institutes of Health (NIH). (2010, January). *Definitions of criteria and considerations for K critiques.* Retrieved from http://grants.nih.gov/grants/peer/critiques/k.htm

National Institutes of Health (NIH). (2014, November). *SF424 (R&R) Application Guide for NIH and Other PHS agencies.* Retrieved from http://grants.nih.gov/grants/funding/424/SF424_RR_Guide_General_VerC.pdf

TRANSLATIONAL RESEARCH, EVIDENCE-BASED PRACTICE, AND DEMONSTRATION PROJECT PROPOSALS

TRANSLATIONAL RESEARCH

Purpose and Structure

Translational research is designed to get interventions that work to the people who need them, to get people to do what we know they should do, or to get providers to do what we know they need to do. Translational projects are essential because a lot of interventions that research has shown to be efficacious are never put into practice and, therefore, no one benefits from them.

There are three types of translational projects, and the first two are generally considered research. Some are designed to move interventions that have been found efficacious into general practice. For example, a project might focus on establishing routine use in health departments of an intervention found to reduce depression among low-income pregnant women. The original research may have been conducted in a health department, but the study paid for expert interveners to provide these women with care. The goal of the translational project is to enable women to get this care in the health department without the need for extra funding. So the project might include finding a way for health department staff to provide the intervention as a part of existing programs. A translational project designed to make a Centers for Disease Control and Prevention (CDC)-approved diabetes self-care management intervention broadly available might involve developing community sites for the intervention, and training lay health workers to provide the intervention. Or a translational project to increase the duration of breastfeeding might involve training staff in

157

business offices and production facilities to enable women to pump breast milk during breaks at work. These projects are research projects, and they are often funded by the National Institutes of Health (NIH) and other major agencies; therefore, a proposal for funding such a project needs to be written like the standard research proposal.

A second kind of translational project is designed to get patients and the rest of us to do what we need to do. Much of this research is intervention research focused on individual behavior change, and it is also translational research, whether it is called that or not. That is, research has already made it clear what people should do to protect their health or to manage their disease—do not smoke, do not drink too much, eat right, exercise, check your blood sugar, take your medicines when you are supposed to, and so forth. However, we all know that many people do not do what they are supposed to do. For example, people with heart failure need to follow a low-sodium diet to avoid fluid accumulation, and they need to weigh themselves every day to check on fluid accumulation. But most people with heart failure do not do either. As a result, they experience worsening symptoms and often must be hospitalized to deal with them. Thus, many interventions are designed to persuade, encourage, assist, support, and engage people in doing the things they need to do to protect their health or manage disease.

Writing the Proposal

Both of these types of translational research proposals are generally submitted for funding and they need to be written like standard NIH proposals; they will be reviewed using the same criteria. Therefore, we recommend that you follow the suggestions for writing an NIH proposal provided in Chapter 5. To begin, you need to develop the rationale for the study, based on the literature. The general steps in reviewing the literature are summarized in Chapter 2, which tells you how to find, read, analyze, and report the work done on the problem. Your task is to follow those steps and fit them into your situation and proposed project.

If you are doing translational research to move an efficacious intervention into general practice, begin by identifying the problem and the difficulties in solving it in practice, then review the literature on the interventions that have been tried and discuss their successes and shortcomings. Next describe your intervention and its efficacy, and then use the literature to describe approaches to putting such an intervention into broad practice, say in physicians' offices, or perhaps public health departments. Finally, identify the approach you have chosen and indicate why it has greater potential for success than other approaches tried. The organization of this rationale is like that of any other research proposal.

The methods will also be described as in an NIH proposal. However, these projects also involve issues that do not arise in typical research. For example, if you plan to implement an intervention in community settings using lay health workers, you must find organizations or agencies that are willing to take on the job of intervening with community members and then you must develop relationships with these agencies so that you have their trust and their commitment to serve people. Your proposal must also provide convincing evidence that this approach will be sustainable after the funding ends; thus, the commitment of community agencies must include a commitment to ongoing training of lay health workers to carry out the intervention. If you plan to write this type of proposal, it is wise to begin making community contacts long before you plan to submit the proposal.

If you are doing translational research to engage individuals in following a healthier diet, exercising as they should, or better managing their disease or disability, first identify the problem, next briefly discuss the other efforts that have been made to get people to make the change you are focusing on, and point out their successes and shortcomings. Finally, focus on your approach and provide good evidence of its greater potential for success.

In describing your methods, again, follow the organization of any other research proposal. However, these projects, such as projects designed to move efficacious interventions into general practice, must also address issues that are not involved in standard research. For example, if you plan to try a new approach to getting older African American women with diabetes to follow a tested diabetes self-management program, you must think about where you can do this, whether the community can be engaged in ensuring that these women are recruited for an intervention program, who will ensure that the women can access the intervention, who will carry out the intervention, and what the possibilities are for sustainability if the study finds the approach efficacious. If you plan to try an intervention that is designed to improve health literacy in low-income parents of children with asthma, you need to be able to access these parents, ensure that they have access to information and support, and offer suggestions for continuing the program after funding ends. Proposals for this type of research should, therefore, focus on issues in implementation and maintenance.

EVIDENCE-BASED PRACTICE PROJECTS

Purpose and Structure

A third type of translational research is designed to get practitioners to do what they need to do; this type of research is generally thought of as evidence-based practice (EBP) change, and is not usually funded by major agencies, though there are exceptions. EBP projects focus on providers; they are designed to improve care delivery; that is, they are quality improvement projects. Distinctions between quality improvement and EBP projects are a bit fuzzy and slippery though people are often adamant about these distinctions; therefore, it may be wise to avoid labeling your project as one or the other. It is particularly important to avoid the label of quality improvement since sometimes people look down on quality improvement efforts and say they do not qualify as research. Indeed, a quality improvement project for which the design and methods are so weak that the findings are not credible would not qualify as translational research. And a project that has no relevance for anyone other than the individuals whose behavior it is designed to change in your organization would not be considered research, because it would not be applicable to others—and, therefore, no one needs to be told about it. However, quality improvement efforts are in most cases designed to solve problems that many people or agencies experience and thus are EBP projects. For example, many hospitals see frequent hospitalizations of heart failure patients because the patients have not kept their sodium intake low enough. A project designed to engage nurses in effectively teaching patients with heart failure, and their family caregivers how to assess the amount of sodium in the foods they eat, is attacking a problem that is common and the solution of which would benefit both patients and hospitals. Projects such as this are prime examples of EBP projects that offer a way to translate study findings into real-world actions.

Some people draw a distinction between research and EBP projects, and indeed, research is designed to provide new information about problems or develop and test new solutions to problems, whereas EBP projects are designed to translate research findings into existing practice. But the distinction between research and translational research is fuzzy, and therefore, if you plan to do an EBP project, it is wise to learn as much about research methods as you can, because if you understand how to conduct research, your project will be stronger and your outcomes more likely to be credible and useful to others.

EBP projects are intervention projects: You are intervening to improve practice by persuading, encouraging, assisting, supporting, and engaging staff or administrators or policy makers to use the findings of research to do something better or more effectively or efficiently. Many hospitals are encouraging staff to conduct EBP projects to improve the efficiency and effectiveness of care. Also, while the requirements of Doctor of Nursing Practice (DNP) programs vary, many require students to conduct an EBP project as a capstone or final assignment. The short-term goals of the capstone EBP project are to improve practice in a particular hospital or other agency and to disseminate the findings to similar agencies or practices. The long-term goal is to learn how to propose and carry out evidence-based projects so that you can continue to do these projects and teach other staff to do them and thus help to improve practice wherever you are. It is important to remember this long-term goal in both proposing and carrying out a capstone project. Some DNP students write capstone proposals that are almost like PhD dissertation proposals, and some programs even call them dissertations. But you are not going to be able to write proposals like that in practice or teach other people to write proposals like that. Further, the traditional dissertation proposal is much too long, and the organization is fragmented and thus not useful for developing a concise, coherent project. And using this organization will make it extremely difficult for you to develop an article reporting your work, even if it was highly successful. (Also, it takes an inordinate amount of faculty time to read—time that could be better spent in helping you think.) Therefore, we do not recommend that you write an EBP project like a traditional dissertation. It is better to learn to write a proposal that is concise but clear, provides the rationale for the project but does not go into lengthy details about all the research, carefully describes the methods you will use to improve practice, provides evidence of the likelihood of success of your proposed project, and offers a model for others to follow. This is not only a logical way to proceed, but it will also provide you a coherent basis for writing an article on the project once it is complete, and a useful template for doing more proposals for EBP projects. If your school's guidelines are more complex, you might ask if you can do this shorter form and provide whatever additional information your committee wants in another form such as an appendix.

Writing the Proposal

The most effective approach is to organize the proposal in three sections: the rationale or need for the project, the project methods and, more briefly, the plans for analysis and dissemination. Follow the suggestions given in Chapter 2 on the rationale for a study, and in Chapter 3 on methods. You should be able to write a compelling proposal in 20 to 30 pages maximum; that is the length necessary for proposals for funding, and proposals for your agency, so this gives you practice in developing proposals that will succeed. (If you have written an extensive literature review, you should take it out of the proposal and think about publishing it as a review paper.) This organization will also help you move toward publication since once you finish, you will have a draft of everything except the findings and discussion already on paper.

The Rationale for the Project

Whether you are developing an EBP project in your agency or a capstone project for the DNP, writing the proposal involves many of the steps you would follow in developing any research proposal. To begin, you must make the case for the study, or the rationale for doing it. As we noted in Chapter 2, the rationale or argument for any study has four parts. In developing EBP projects, the four parts are: (a) There is a problem in the delivery of health care; (b) research has provided a solution to the problem, that is, the evidence to be put into practice; but (c) the solution has not been tried in practice, or the solution has not been tried in some settings where it is needed, or efforts to implement the solution have not been fully successful; and therefore; (d) we are going to implement the solution where it is needed, or implement it in a way that will succeed in changing practice.

If you are proposing an EBP project, the proposal will be a little different from standard research proposals. To develop a proposal, you must first identify a problem in the delivery or organization of health care. What have you seen in your work that is problematic? Are hospitalized patients not getting enough information about how to take care of an incision when they go home? Are the children coming to a school health clinic not getting enough help in managing their chronic diseases? Are new first-time mothers not getting enough instruction and support to successfully breastfeed? Are patients spending too much time in the emergency department (ED) before they are admitted to the hospital? Is the Rapid Response Team not being used? Are experienced nurses bullying new, inexperienced nurses? What is the problem as you have observed it? Do its effects matter? And can you solve it?

When identifying a problem, it is essential to focus on something that is both important and soluble, otherwise you will be wasting your time. So even though the first step in developing an EBP project is identifying a problem, at the same time you need to be thinking about the methods you will use to solve it. We described the methods of a study in detail in Chapter 3 and we describe some particular methods needed for EBP projects later in this chapter, but do not wait to begin thinking about methods. Start now

The ideal setting for an EBP project is your place of employment. You know the problems there, you know the people, and you know the challenges to making practice change, and the ways to deal with those challenges. In some other setting you could be at a loss. So plan to make change in your institution or agency, whether this is an agency-backed project or a DNP proposal. Another point to remember: When you are deciding on a problem to tackle, focus on something you care about. Carrying out a project is difficult, but it is even more difficult if it does not really interest you. It is often helpful to begin by making a list of possible problems to study in your setting; then you can talk about them to others in the setting to help you decide which problem is most important to study now, most interesting to you, and most likely to be something you can solve.

Once you have identified a problem, the next step is to find out what is known about the problem in general. Most DNP students and most practitioners have no difficulty identifying specific problems that need attention in their unit, on their floor, in their agency or practice. And those specializing in education have no difficulty identifying problems in educating undergraduates (and graduate students for that matter). But in order for your work to be applicable to others, you have to show that the problem you see is also experienced by others. That is the first reason why you review the literature—to see whether others have the problem. When you begin the literature review, first make a list of words that describe the practice problem you wish to solve. Let us say you have observed that elderly patients sometimes develop delirium after surgery as a result of the drugs given to them to prevent nausea and vomiting from narcotics. Think about the words that will help you find articles on this topic—"delirium" combined with "surgery," "hospitalized elderly," "elderly" combined with "surgery," "narcotic allergies" combined with "surgery," "elderly" combined with "delirium," and so forth. Then using these words, identify and review the literature in these areas to see what others are saying about the problem.

Always focus on the literature in your area. For example, if the problem you are interested in is delays in the ED, look at the literature on ED management, ED operations, triage in the ED, delays in moving patients, patient satisfaction with ED services, and so forth, to see if others are experiencing this problem. Or if you find that at your health department clinic you are seeing a lot of low-income women with postpartum depression, check the literature on depression in pregnant women and postpartum women to see if others are also seeing this—to ensure that this is not unique to your clinic. In reviewing the literature, you will probably find that others have also seen the problem your agency is experiencing. Thus your problem is a general problem, not limited to your site. This is key to ensuring that your work will be applicable to others.

In addition, by reviewing the literature you may discover that other people report problems that you have not thought of, but may well be experiencing also. Thus, the literature helps you think more broadly about problems in your organization and learn about possible solutions.

Sometimes, because many practitioners do not report what they know about problems in practice, you may find little in the literature about your particular problem. Nevertheless, you will certainly see something in the literature about its consequences, and you can extrapolate from those. For example, you may have observed that some practitioners in your organization resist working with others as equals. You may not find much in the literature about resistance to working as equals with others, but you will see numerous articles about the negative consequences of health care hierarchies and the need for better communication and teamwork. So you note the negative outcomes others have observed and report what others have said about their causes, and you can also suggest that resistance may be a part of the problem.

In reviewing the literature to discover whether others have the same practice problems you have, it is important to recognize that some of the information you find may be anecdotal data or opinions. While the best evidence comes from rigorous research, in looking for reports of practice issues, you may not find much of that. Nevertheless, people's opinions about the importance of a problem and their clinical observations of the problem may be sufficient for you to conclude that, indeed, this is a problem for others, not just you.

Once you have established the existence of the problem, you want to look at what people have already done about the problem. Have researchers found a way to assess the elderly for risk of delirium? Have they suggested effective ways to deal with nausea and vomiting in elderly patients postsurgery? Have staff in orthopedic units been taught to use these effective approaches, and are they using them? Or not?

As you check the literature on solutions, it is important to focus primarily on research. While opinions and anecdotal data can be helpful in establishing the broad existence of a problem, they do not give you reliable evidence about a solution, though they may be suggestive. As you analyze studies, you may conclude that while some interventions have had effects, they were not very strong. It is important to figure out why they have not been more effective, so you can avoid the problems those authors had and institute a solution that is effective. What methods did the authors use? What did the authors say about reasons for lack of effectiveness? And what do you think? This is how you develop the argument for trying a new intervention that has greater potential for success.

For example, if your interest is in assessing risk for postpartum depression in low-income women seen at the health clinic, you may discover from the literature that many women who suffer postpartum depression have been found to show early signs of risk. Further, some researchers have found that if these women are assessed during pregnancy and made aware of risk, they can avoid acute problems and get treatment if they need it. And there is an instrument available to assess risk of depression. Thus, the research has both documented the existence of the problem and provided a solution to the problem, that is, the evidence that needs to be translated into practice.

If someone has also reported an intervention that was effective in getting providers to use this instrument to assess pregnant women for risk of postpartum depression, you do not need to develop an intervention to change your practice; you just need to use the one already in the literature. But if no intervention has been effective in getting staff to assess these women, you have a reason for developing and testing such an intervention. If an intervention has been tried with staff in high-end specialty practices seeing well-off women, but not with the low-income women you see, you may need to adapt the intervention for clinic staff caring for low-income women. The key is to recognize that there is evidence of a solution: the research has shown that assessing women for depression during pregnancy, using an instrument found to be valid and reliable, helps to prevent postpartum depression. It is also important to show that the evidence has not been translated into practice in settings like yours and, therefore, your project is designed to do just that.

Thus, whatever your problem, the argument for your study will be this: There is a problem in health (e.g., postpartum depression, which exists not only in your practice but in many practices), some work has been done on the problem (research shows that it helps to assess women for risk and increase their awareness of risk and there is an available instrument for assessing risk), but the work has not gone far enough (no intervention has been reported that is effective in getting staff to assess low-income pregnant women for risk) and, therefore, an intervention needs to be developed to ensure that staff make these assessments.

Whatever the guidelines for a capstone project at your university, or whatever the guidelines for developing EBP in your agency or institution, this is the logic for an EBP project. It is extremely useful to outline what you will propose using this logic, as follows:

1. The broad problem in the delivery of health care as reported in the literature.
2. The problem as observed in your practice (your unit, agency, institution).
3. Solutions to the problem shown by research to be effective, which is the evidence to be put into practice.
4. Interventions tried to date to implement the solution—moving from the general to the particular and ending with interventions tried in settings most like yours.
5. Shortcomings of these existing interventions for your situation (they may have been used with a different type of provider, or in a different type of setting, or there were difficulties noted in implementing the intervention or assessing its effects).
6. Purpose of the proposed study.

Before you write this last section, it is extremely helpful to make a detailed outline of your points, using the aforementioned logic. Then show the outline to colleagues (or advisors) and ask them if you have made a compelling case for your project. They can help you see where there are holes in your logic and you need to be clearer about the rationale for the project. When you begin to write, use the outline headings as topic sentences and fit the information you have under each. When you describe the literature, always start with general information and then move to more specific data in particular studies. Review articles, which provide a summary of the research to date, can be very helpful in showing you how to organize your review. However, reviews may include studies on the importance of the problem as well as studies reporting interventions to solve the problem, and you need to separate those. Describe work on the problem first, then solutions, then the need for a workable solution in practice.

Some DNP programs require you to have a conceptual framework for your EBP project (most hospitals and other agencies will not require this). If your intervention was actually developed based on a conceptual framework, then present it here, at the end of the argument for your study. However, you may have developed your approach based on your reasoning about how to proceed. In that case, do not include a conceptual framework, unless you are required to have one. If you must present a conceptual framework, remember that this project is about putting evidence into practice—it is not about developing evidence. So you do not want a framework that shows how you develop an intervention; you want a framework about the process of putting interventions into practice—about making practice change.

Proposed Methods

Once you have developed the rationale for intervening to translate research evidence into practice, you must describe the methods you propose to implement your intervention. In EBP projects, you are proposing to get practitioners or administrators or policy makers to use research to guide what they do. In writing your proposal, you need to follow the standard methods of research as closely as possible. (These are described in detail in Chapter 3.) However, you also need to show that the methods you plan are doable in your setting and will also be doable by others—or you will not have anything to tell others. For example, if you propose to help providers adequately assess the physical problems of patients with mental illness, but this strategy requires medical expertise, then you can hardly expect it to be used in mental health clinics where there is no physician or nurse practitioner. Similarly, if you propose to use a new assessment tool for delirium in the hospitalized elderly and you expect staff nurses to use this new tool, the tool better not be complicated or lengthy—or no one in the real world will have time to use it.

When deciding on methods, it is important to remember that researchers often have the funding to employ staff to carry out an intervention and collect data, but you may not. Agencies likes the Agency for Healthcare Research and Quality (AHRQ) and the CDC fund some EBP projects, but most DNP students and many clinicians doing EBP in their agencies will not have funding. Researchers have this funding because they must ensure that their protocol is rigorously followed and the data are accurate—otherwise the findings will not be credible. When you do EBP projects, you also need to carry out and monitor your intervention rigorously for the same reasons, but often the best you can hope for is some in-kind support from the hospital or agency. Sometimes, the best you can get is verbal support or a letter recommending your work. Therefore, you have to think very carefully about how you will get this done.

The first thing to think about is this: If you want to get staff to change their practice, your methods need to include strategies for involving staff in the change. Ordering staff is far less effective than engaging them. One way of engaging them is to consult with them from the beginning. Take a lesson from community-based participatory research, in which the community provides input into problem identification, planning and implementation—with the idea that their involvement throughout the process makes change more likely to occur and more likely to last. You will also find that involvement of staff in EBP projects helps to expand interest in and understanding of evidence and its importance: people who are involved in translating research into practice learn about it, become interested in it, and often move on to develop more evidence based projects and also research.

If you plan to change hospital or agency practice, you will need the support of administrators and to get this, you must show a convincing reason for change. The basic reasons for changing practice are that the change improves care without increasing costs, or the change cuts costs but does not reduce the quality of care. Sometimes you may need to make the argument that change will improve care at an increased cost, but the cost will be offset by savings down the line. For example, home visits by physicians or nurse practitioners may improve care but they also cost more; however, over time they may lead to huge savings through keeping elderly people independent and at home, instead of sending them to a nursing home. Currently, such arguments are most persuasive in accountable care organizations, but they may become more broadly convincing over time.

Sometimes to change their practice, staff simply need to be made aware of a problem or reminded of its importance; sometimes all they need is an information session on what to do about it. Thus, many EBP projects involve some kind of in-service education or training, whether individually, in staff meetings, or online. Such projects are often evaluated by collecting data before the intervention to determine the extent to which staff understand what they should be doing, then doing the teaching, and finally, collecting data again after the intervention to see if there are improvements in staff's knowledge and perhaps their willingness to do what is needed. These are the simplest EBP projects. But even a simple project can be challenging. Before you implement a practice change, you may need to present a proposal to the agency's institutional review board (IRB). And if you are doing a capstone project, you may need to send a proposal to the university's IRB. (It is wise to do that even if it is not required, because without IRB approval, you may find it difficult to publish your findings.) Also, if you plan to do an intervention on agency time, you must have the approval of administrators or managers. Further, you need to show them the potential utility of the project, because if they do not like what you plan to do, you will find it very difficult to carry out your plans. Also, many larger hospitals and health care organizations have research committees that have to review and approve a proposal before it can be carried out in the organization, whether it is using staff or patients.

And if you are going to talk to every staff person individually, you have to find the time to do so and you have to find times when they can talk to you. If you are going to teach people in a staff meeting, you have to schedule a time for it, and you have to make sure everyone in every shift will be there or find a way to give a makeup session or talk to the absentees individually. If you teach online, you have to find a way to determine whether all the staff completed the session, and on and on.

Then, to examine improvements in knowledge and perhaps attitudes, you will need a questionnaire that assesses these, and if none are available, you need to develop one. It is important to think through what you are trying to change with your intervention so that your questionnaire collects useful data. You can sometimes take a questionnaire on another topic and modify it for your topic. But if you use someone else's questionnaire, you may need to get permission, unless it is in the public domain. Also, that questionnaire may have established validity and reliability, but if you change it much, they are not maintained, so you may need to test them again. If you develop your own questionnaire, you will not have any data showing that it is valid and reliable. But you can at least ask a group of experts to examine it for content validity before you use the questionnaire and amend it based on their suggestions. It is always helpful to have on hand a research text book (perhaps you can buy back the one you sold after your last research course) because this will help you with such things as questionnaire development and other research issues. Use the text like a recipe book: when you have a problem, check the index for the right recipe.

The goal of an EBP intervention is for staff to do more of what they need to do after the intervention than before—complete more assessments or provide patients more information or relieve pain more effectively, and so on. Your project may simply assess improvements in knowledge, not improvements in practice and, if so, you need to be clear about that. You may be assuming that with more knowledge or skill, practitioners will improve practice. But do not suggest that your intervention will improve practice because you would not be able to show that. More complicated projects not only assess knowledge and skills but actually assess actions after an intervention, but these may require more involvement of staff and more data collection. If, for example, you want staff to routinely assess hospitalized elderly patients for delirium or you want nursing home staff to assist residents to eat instead of feeding them, you will need to collect observational or chart data on what staff do before your teaching, then collect similar data after the intervention to see whether staff have changed their practice. And you may need to collect those data not just once but over a period of time to see whether the change becomes routine and endures. You may also want to collect data on staff in another similar unit who do not receive the intervention to provide a comparison that helps to show whether your intervention is useful. Finally, if you want to determine whether a change in actions by providers is related to a change in patient outcomes, you need to collect data not just on what providers do but on what happens to patients.

The question is what data do you need? It is important to think this through so that you do not discover at the end of the project that you missed something crucial for understanding your outcomes. How many people are eligible for the practice change intervention? Will they be required to participate or is this voluntary? Do they need to provide informed consent to participate in the intervention or, if required, in the evaluation of the intervention? If so, how many do you expect to consent? What are the characteristics of these staff—age, education, experience, and so forth? Will you collect those data? Do these characteristics differ from the staff who do not participate? How will you know? What about staff in a comparison unit, if you have one? And what exactly do you expect staff to learn about and then do? Will all of that be adequately covered in your teaching intervention? What will you observe before and after the intervention?

If you plan to observe change in practice, will you be able to observe staff without altering their behavior through the very act of observing? Will the chart show you what you need? If you have a comparison group from another similar unit who do not receive the intervention, will you collect the same data from these people? With consent? When will you collect the data and how? What incentive will they have to participate? And will you have permission from their unit manager?

To describe your methods, use the organization and the list of items that we suggest in Chapter 3 for almost any proposal. However, take these suggestions knowing that you cannot do everything with the rigor of say, an NIH proposal, and you must also deal with the realities of your situation. Thus, some things will not be included in your proposal (e.g., you may not be able to fully monitor the fidelity of the intervention), but there will be other things in your proposal that are not usually included in a research proposal (e.g., steps in obtaining support from administrators and ensuring participation of all staff in the teaching).

Plans for Analysis

Finally, as in any research proposal, talk about what you will do with the data. How will you analyze the information you collect? What will you describe? What comparisons will you make—for example, before and after data? If you plan to administer a questionnaire, will you look only at the total score or also at individual items? Will you compare participants and non-participants? Will you compare participants with different levels of education or experience? Perhaps you will compare participants with a group on another unit who do not receive the intervention? In that case, will you have enough participants to test the significance of differences between your intervention group and a comparison group? (It is not likely if the intervention is unit based because the n's are 1 and 1.) Most EBP projects have small samples and, therefore, your analysis is unlikely to be complex. Probably you will simply need to state what comparisons you will make and how you will do them. You want to tell readers what you plan to do with the data, and you always want to indicate your plan to publish the work.

Notes on Writing

If you are not accustomed to writing proposals and feel terror about describing and critiquing the literature, it is useful to remember that you have major skills that are essential to good writing: skill in observing and skill in making decisions. All nurses have these clinical skills; the key is to recognize that good writing is also about observing and making decisions. You are expert at observing clinical problems—and now you are observing and describing a problem in your agency; in the articles you read, you observe what others said about the problem, and you make decisions about how well those others understood the problem and how good their solutions were. Then you make decisions about what to include in your description of what these others have done. Finally, you present your decision to try something new. Thus, you are not moving into a totally different world when you begin to write; rather, you are translating your skills in the clinical area to another area of operation.

DEMONSTRATION PROJECTS

Demonstration projects are not considered research, and most agencies funding them do not want research: They want a solution to a problem that is important and widespread. Your project is expected to demonstrate that solution, not just for your situation, but also for your state or region or the nation. But just to be clear: Funding agencies expect you to evaluate the success of your project, and evaluation is a type of research. So even if you never use the word research, if your methods are rigorous, you will be able to publish your findings, and indeed, the agency will want you to publish as a way of disseminating your solution to the problem.

Most funding agencies have guidelines that tell you how they want you to write a proposal for demonstration projects, but those guidelines vary; some want a proposal written in a series of small boxes in which you provide answers to specific questions; some want a proposal that is almost like a research proposal; some want you to write a brief letter of intent first, and if they like it, they will ask for a full proposal. (Incidentally, it is much harder to write a brief proposal than a full proposal, so you need to work really hard at this early version.) Many foundations want the kind of proposal we suggest in the following.

First, indicate the need for the project you are proposing. Use the literature to establish the importance of the problem, then provide data on the extent of the problem nationally and regionally, and perhaps in your state, as well as your location. Next give the purpose of your proposed project. Here you may want to provide specific aims or objectives. For example, if you are proposing a school-based project to prevent or reduce obesity in children, what exactly do you plan to do? Your objectives might include providing workshops for teachers on ways to increase physical activity among students without requiring additional time, and workshops for parents on providing foods with fewer calories, as well as consultations with the cafeteria staff on ways to reduce calories. You might also offer sessions for students on avoiding sugary drinks and fatty foods, and exercising more. If this is a multi-year project, list your aims by year. Think through what you need to do when. For example, you probably would not do workshops for teachers every year, though you probably will do sessions for students every year and you may hold sessions for new teachers every year.

If your project is intended to demonstrate a way to provide low-income urban residents better access to nutritious foods, your aims might include developing a farmers' market in the area you plan to serve, or working with the city parks and recreation department to develop a community garden and helping residents learn to grow gardens. You might also plan to help interested individuals turn a part of their yards into small gardens and provide plowing and seeds.

Next describe the population you plan to serve and the number of participants you expect. Is your school-based project designed for students in all grades? Elementary grades? Will it be for all students in the grades you target? How many students? If your plan is to increase access to better foods for low-income residents, what area of your town or city will you target? Why that particular area? How many people live in that area? And how many do you expect to participate?

Then describe the methods you will use to recruit participants for your project. If this is a community-based project, will you use flyers? Distributed where? Are there agencies that will help you recruit? What are they? How will they recruit? Will you ask people who have agreed to participate to recruit others?

After describing your population and expected participants and the ways you will get these participants, describe the activities you plan to carry out in order to achieve the aims or objectives of your project. For example, if you plan workshops to teach gardening to low-income residents of a particular area in your city, where will you hold the workshops? When? Who will sponsor them? What will the workshops include? How long will they last? Who will conduct them? How will you get people there and get them home afterward? Will you provide refreshments? If you plan to develop a farmers' market in the area, what activities will be necessary to bring this about? Think through all the things you need to do to achieve each of your objectives and list them here.

Implementation of projects in the community is always more difficult than conducting a controlled trial—because the real world gets in the way. People disappear, or they have to work when a workshop is being held, or they cannot get their landlord's permission to plow a part of the yard for a garden. The people who run the local farmers' market cannot find an appropriate space for a market in the area you are targeting, and the parks and recreation people do not have a space for a community garden. You need to factor these possibilities into your methods; for example, you might offer makeup sessions for participants who cannot get there for the first offering. If you plan carefully and think ahead, you have a good chance of successfully carrying out this project.

After describing your planned activities, describe your plans for evaluating the success of the demonstration. What data do you need to collect? Clearly you will want data on the number of people who agree to participate in your project and the number who complete it. This is essential: If you cannot get participants, you will waste the funding agency's money. You also need to record information on how activities are conducted, whether those who participate think they are useful, and what the outcomes are. For example, if you plan to help those attending a homeless shelter get care for their feet, what do you expect to happen? Will you check feet, provide care, then check them again? How? When? Think about indicators of success and then decide how you will collect data on those indicators.

Finally, for any demonstration project you must talk about sustainability. Foundations and other agencies do not like to give you money for a project that will end when the money ends. Your goal is to develop something that can be maintained without external funding. For example, will the school take over doing workshops for parents to help them improve nutrition at home, perhaps at parent–teacher meetings? Can you get a commitment from the people who run the cafeteria to continue efforts to reduce calories and fat in the foods they serve? If you are starting a program to care for people at the homeless shelter, can the shelter staff provide this care? If not, is there a local university whose students will provide care as part of clinical experiences? You cannot say, "We will seek funding to continue the program." You must show the funding agency that the program will continue, and you must produce commitments to that effect. One last thing—you should include your plans to disseminate your findings, not only in published articles for professionals, but also in presentations for local people and others who might be interested in replicating the project. You want to offer to make available materials that could help them. This is how you change the world.

NINE

EDUCATIONAL TRAINING GRANT PROPOSALS

Educational training programs focus on producing health professionals with specific types of expertise. Thus, educational training grant proposals are written primarily to fund the education of particular groups of providers, for example, psychiatric mental health nurses, nurse anesthetists, physician assistants, or physical therapists, or to support the development of new programs, such as PhD programs, Doctor of Nursing Practice (DNP) programs, programs to increase diversity in the health professions, or programs in interprofessional education. While foundations and even some corporations fund educational training programs, most of the funding for these projects comes from workforce agencies or national agencies, and they have relatively standard guidelines.

Educational training projects are not research projects; funding agencies are quite clear about that. But just so you know, a rose by any other name would smell as sweet. In other words, while these projects do not involve research, they do require evaluation and evaluation is a form of research—so if you conduct these projects carefully, you will essentially be doing research, and you will be able to publish your outcomes while also improving the training of professionals and their care of people. Thus, it is important to design your project thoughtfully and carry it out rigorously.

The big funder of educational training grants is the federal Health Resources and Services Administration (HRSA). If you are interested in developing an educational training program, look first at HRSA calls and find out what their priorities are. If you fit one of those priorities, this is the place to go. However, other agencies and foundations also fund educational training, so it is important to look broadly to see where you can find other funding.

The HRSA calls generally come out in the fall. If you plan to write a proposal for HRSA funding, and you have a reasonable idea about what they are interested in, it is important to begin developing a proposal without waiting for the call—HRSA does not give you much time, so you need to get ahead of the game. Generally, HRSA allows you a total of 80 pages for everything related to the grant proposal, including the budget, bio-sketches of faculty who will be involved, and all the other supplementary materials. Many of these can be developed ahead of time, leaving you essential time for developing the proposal narrative. Here we will focus on the narrative, but do not forget all that other information. Your proposal will be thrown out if you do not include it. Also, before beginning, note the HRSA review criteria for training grant proposals: There are currently six criteria. The first of these is Purpose and Need, which includes addressing national, regional, and local needs; needs related to the primary care workforce in the community; needs for diversity; and ways in which the proposed project will address these needs. The second criterion is Response to Program Purpose, which includes providing an appropriate work plan, methods, and resolution of challenges. The work plan needs to describe the project timeline, stakeholders, and the people to be served, as well as clear and comprehensive goals, objectives and sub-objectives, with plans for achieving these. Methods should include clear narrative descriptions of strategies for achieving the project objectives, and the section Resolution of Challenges should show understanding of potential obstacles and challenges to achievement of the objectives along with resources and plans for overcoming these. The third review criterion is Impact, which includes evaluation and technical support capacity and project sustainability. The fourth criterion is Organizational Information, Resources, and Capabilities, in which you describe the capacity of your organization and staff to successfully carry out the project. The fifth criterion is Support Requested, which involves showing that your proposed budget is reasonable for every year of the project. Finally, the sixth criterion is Program-Specific Criteria, which involves showing that you will carry out the particular program you are proposing over the project period and address evidence-based models of integrated care. Particular calls will provide more specific information about what you need to do to meet each of these criteria, and some calls may have additional criteria. So read the call with great care and keep the criteria in mind as you develop your proposal.

The narrative should begin with an introduction. Next comes a needs assessment, then a description of the target population and the methods you plan to use to conduct the project, along with a description of how you plan to evaluate the project. You need to indicate what impact you expect the project to have and to provide organizational information including project personnel, the plan for recruiting or assigning faculty to the training project, consultants, the capabilities of your organization, technical support available, community support, and linkages with other organizations. This should be followed with a detailed work plan, and finally, a description of how you plan to ensure the sustainability and replicability of the project and what its impact will be. Whew! A lot, but you can do it.

INTRODUCTION

The Introduction is actually an executive summary or a long abstract: It introduces the problem that your project is designed to solve; gives a quick needs assessment, including data on the target population and pool of potential applicants; describes the purpose of your project; indicates how the project is innovative and how the training it provides will improve health care, and/or health outcomes for patients, families or communities; and then describes your proposed methods and the capacity of your organization to carry out the project. The Introduction generally concludes with a brief description of how you will evaluate the success of the program. While there is no specific page limit for the Introduction, it should be brief—both because you have an overall page limit that will look more and more difficult to meet as you go along, and because your readers want a summary, not a long description that contains the same information that will appear in the coming pages. Your aim is to give reviewers a concise, compelling argument for funding this project. The most efficient way to do this is to write this section after you have written the proposal. As we have noted elsewhere, it is much easier to summarize something you have already written than to summarize a story that is still in your head. So before writing this, construct the major sections of the proposal narrative.

NEED

This section is crucial. If you cannot provide strong evidence of need, you have no case for funding. Therefore, begin by describing the problem you are going to solve. It is important to first point out that this is a broad problem, not simply a problem for you: An educational training project should be a model for solving a problem nationally or at least regionally, not just in your town or your institution. There is no lack of problems in health care that might be resolved or at least mitigated by training of more health care professionals. But you must document the importance of the particular problem you will address. You can follow the guides to developing the rationale for a study that we provide in Chapter 2, but do not get carried away by the literature: you want data, data, data.

For example, if you plan to train psychiatric-mental health nurses for work in rural areas, the argument for your training program begins with the statement that in many rural areas there are few providers of mental health services though mental health problems are widespread. To document this, provide some data on the state of mental health care in the nation: How many people have mental health problems, how many of these live in rural areas, and how many are not getting the care they need? Then move to your region or state: What proportion of the population lives in rural areas? What kinds of mental health needs exist for this group? How many of them are not receiving adequate mental health care? Is this related to rural location or to poverty, minority race, or ethnicity?

You then need to point to the importance of psychiatric-mental health nurses for improving access to care. Note that often psychiatric-mental health nurses are the only specialists in mental health services available in rural areas, but there are too few of these psychiatric-mental health nurses. To document this, provide the data. How many psychiatric-mental health nurse practitioners are practicing in your state? How many in rural or underserved areas? How many would be needed to ensure good access to mental health care? How many of these nurses are being prepared each year? How many of them are going into rural areas? Your aim is to show that these nurses are essential for providing mental health care in rural areas, but too few are being trained, especially from rural areas and, therefore, we need a new training program to increase their numbers.

If you are interested in a diversity grant, first you need to remind readers of the need for a diverse health care workforce, one that reflects the large and growing populations of African Americans and Hispanics in many states (and Asians in some states). You might note that when providers share some of the experiences and characteristics of patients (and sometimes language), this helps to build trust and understanding and makes providers more sensitive to patients (reference your statements). Then note that the numbers of African American and Hispanic or Asian nurses in the nation are abysmally low. Provide data, with references to document this. Then you need some figures about your state or region: What proportion of the population is African American or Hispanic (or whatever group you are interested in)? Do health care providers share any of their experiences or characteristics? What proportion of the health professional workforce in your area (nursing, medicine, etc.) is from this race or ethnicity? How many are considering nursing school or medical school each year? Do guidance counselors point them to health professions? How many are applying, and how many are actually being admitted to health professional schools each year? How many are graduating? What factors appear to lead to failure to apply to these programs and failure to complete the programs? What proportion of those who graduate pass licensing examinations? How many are practicing in the areas of greatest need? These are the kinds of figures that make a compelling case for preparing more minority professionals. But you have to dig them out. And present them with references to your sources.

The best way to organize this section is to begin with national data, then discuss the situation in your state or region, and conclude with a description of the problem in your local area and the need for an innovative approach to solve the problem. In this way, you show that this is everybody's concern—not just yours—and you will present a model solution that will be sustainable in your area and can be used by others as well.

You may not always be able to find the data you need to support establishment of a new program. In that case, you may want to do a needs assessment yourself. But remember, if you plan to use the data in a proposal to HRSA, you must conduct this needs assessment well before the call comes out or you won't get the information in time. You can also rely on anecdotal data about need and the opinions of experts in the area, though this kind of information is generally considered less credible than objective data. However, if you think carefully about why this program is important, you should be able to come up with compelling reasons. (Otherwise, why are you doing it?)

Once you have established the problem, you should clearly state the purpose of your project: "We will develop and implement a master's program to train family nurse practitioners for rural underserved areas in the Northwest." "We will implement a program to increase the numbers of minority students who enroll in and graduate from a BSN program in a Southern state." "We will establish a program that enrolls and graduates more American Indians with bachelor's degrees in a health profession." "We will develop a DNP program that prepares graduates to develop evidence-based practices in the care of the elderly." Will establishment of the program depend on funding? If so, make that clear. If you plan to open the new program whether you are funded or not, you will have to say what the funding will enable you to do that you would otherwise not be able to do. Or why would anyone fund you?

TARGET POPULATION

This section shows who will be targeted for your program and provides evidence that there is a pool of people who would be interested in enrolling in the program. If there are not enough people who want the program, starting it will waste the taxpayers' money and it will be a failure. Who is your target population? African Americans in high schools? Community colleges? Universities? Are you planning to enroll nurses practicing in rural areas who would like advanced training and would then practice in their home area? How do you know they want the program? One way to show that there will be sufficient applicants is to conduct a survey of people who might enroll. For example, you might survey your alumni to see how many would be interested in enrolling in a physician's assistant (PA) program or a DNP program, or you might survey nurses across your state to see how many would be interested in a psychiatric-mental health nursing master's program, or consult high school guidance counselors about the numbers of minority students who might be interested in a health professional program, or survey people with a BA or BS to see how many would enroll in a family nurse practitioner (FNP) program with online courses. You can also assess need by surveying people who attend a local or state conference or continuing education program. An assessment of the potential pool of applicants gives you concrete data on the appeal of the proposed program, and it also shows that you know what you are doing. The assessment should make clear the requirements for enrollment in the program; otherwise you may get responses from people who will not qualify—and then you will have inaccurate information about the pool of applicants.

If you do not have the time or resources to conduct a survey, report the data that have led you to believe people will want to enroll. Have you found that despite the call for increases in the numbers of BSN-prepared minority nurses, you are not seeing increases in the enrollment of minorities in BSN programs? Have you found that people in your area are enrolling in PA programs out of state because there are so few slots in the programs in your state? Is there no occupational therapy program in your area? Think back about why you decided to establish this new program. You can also report anecdotal data; maybe you have heard nurses with a BSN decry the lack of master's programs that are online or that allow clinical experiences in one's own place of work. The key is to show that if you start this program, you will fill its slots. And the more slots you have, the better. It is easier to get funded for a program that will prepare 30 nurse anesthetists over X years than a program that will graduate 10 over those years.

PROGRAM

Once you have established the need for the program and the existence of an applicant pool, you need to describe the program itself. Here you do so in a narrative; later in the proposal you will need to construct a table that shows exactly what you will do when, what the expected outcomes are overall and for each of your specific objectives in each year of the program, and who will determine whether those outcomes are achieved and how. The narrative describes what you will do for whom. Begin with your objectives (sometimes called expected outcomes). What do you hope to achieve and when? Most programs will have three to six objectives—not more. If you have too many, you will look scattered (and will probably be scattered). If you are planning to increase diversity in the professional workforce, how exactly do you plan to do that? What specifically do you hope to achieve?

Your first objective might be to enroll X students in your program from minority backgrounds. The second might be to provide tutorials and other assistance to help these students successfully complete your program. A third objective might be to graduate X number of minority students in Y number of years. What will you do to achieve these objectives? Do you plan to recruit minority students in high schools? What high schools? Who is going to do that, in cooperation with whom? Do you have an agreement with the school system allowing this?

And how are you going to ensure that potential enrollees meet the increasingly stringent criteria for getting into your baccalaureate nursing or PA program? Are you going to provide them some summer course work, say on health care terminology, before they graduate from high school? Will you give them an introduction to nursing or other health professional programs in the first 2 years of their undergraduate program? Begin to think about what you need to do to enroll these students and get them through the program. Are you going to do a joint associate degree–BSN program with a community college? How?

If this is a new program, you will need to show that you have the necessary approvals or permissions to conduct the program. You may need external approvals—for example, a new DNP program must be accredited before you can apply for funding for the program. And you will certainly need approval from your school to establish a new program. You will also need to describe the plan of study. How many credits will be required? What courses will students take? What will those courses include? Have they already been developed? Where and how will they be taught? You will need approval from your school's curriculum committee and the faculty to institute these new courses, so make sure you get those approvals before the last minute. You may need to get institutional review board (IRB) approval for the project (if so, see Chapter 13); and even if you don't, you might want to get that approval because it will make publication of your findings easier—many journals now want IRB approval for any data collected. What clinical agencies will you work with for student practice? What criteria have you used to select these? You should have information on file on the criteria you are using and the agencies you have selected, with letters of support from these agencies.

It is wise to begin making your plans long before the HRSA call comes out. As noted earlier, the call doesn't usually leave a great deal of time for preparation—so the more you think about and plan for your proposal in advance, the more likely you are to make a compelling case that the program is feasible and has potential for success. As you are thinking, make notes, lots of notes, about what you want to achieve and how you can do that. Otherwise you may forget important details. As you make notes, begin developing your budget plans. What will it cost to do the activities you are proposing? These notes will help you decide what activities you can actually afford. When you start writing, first list the program objectives and then describe what you will do to achieve these objectives, remembering what it will cost.

Some writers describe the overall program in the narrative, combining the objectives; others take the objectives one by one and write a narrative about what they will do to achieve each. That may lead to some overlap, but you can eliminate that later. The key is to decide which approach seems to flow best and gives readers a logical sequence of information. You might want to try describing the overall program first, and if that seems confusing, then separate the description by objective. It may be helpful to develop your overall work plan (description to follow) before writing this section, because that will have all the details and show you what needs to be included in the narrative and what can be left out.

We suggest concluding the description of the program with at least a brief paragraph on its potential impact. This is important because HRSA and other funding agencies want to know what difference the project will make. If you plan to prepare psychiatric-mental health nurses to provide care in rural areas of your state, presumably you expect that residents in these areas will have better access to such care, which will improve their lives. If you plan to prepare FNPs to work in the Mississippi Delta, you probably expect these practitioners to improve the care of currently underserved residents. If you plan to develop a new interprofessional education program, you probably expect it to improve the coordination of professional practice and reduce fragmentation. It is important to think about what you want to achieve and make it clear for funders.

EVALUATION

It is essential to have an evaluation plan for any training program you propose. You will need to appoint someone who is expert in evaluation to head your evaluation efforts. The person also needs to have the right kinds of credentials or experience. It is helpful to begin the evaluation section with an overview of the kinds of methods you will use—surveys, observations, figures on enrollment and completion, course evaluations, clinical site evaluations, surveys on technology use and challenges, participant responses to the program, faculty perceptions, clinical site perceptions, and so forth.

Then you need to provide specific information on how you will evaluate achievement of each of your program objectives; these are really expected outcomes said in a different way, but you may also want to list expected outcomes. If, for example, your first objective is to enroll X number of students in an interprofessional education program in Y number of years, the expected outcome is that number. The evaluation is designed to provide data showing whether your objectives (or expected outcomes) are achieved. As your objective is to enroll X number of students, it is obvious that you will need to collect data on the number of students you enroll each year. But you also need to collect other data; for example, you will need a record of all recruitment efforts you make and the number of potential applicants you contact individually and, if possible, the reasons why people do not enroll. Do they not meet enrollment criteria? Can they not afford the program? Do they decide they would prefer some other type of program? Probably another objective will be to graduate X number of these students in Y number of years. You not only need graduation figures, but also need factors in the success of those who graduate and reasons why others fail to finish.

If you plan to hold faculty workshops in order to make faculty more sensitive to minority issues in health professional schools, you will need some indicators of whether the workshops are well attended and well received, and whether people think they become more sensitive after attending. You need to use a questionnaire to collect those data. If you plan to assess faculty's attitudes and behaviors in regard to interprofessional education, you will need to survey faculty before and after involvement in the program, and you may need to ask students about faculty as well.

Evaluations are designed not only to show funders that your program was a success but also to provide data for continuous improvement, so you want to know what goes well and what goes wrong along the way. You will therefore need to set up a system for collecting these data as you go and keeping them. And you will need to describe how you will analyze the data to see what the data mean to you. However, it is important to remember that you will not be able to show cause and effect. For example, you may want to determine the effects of the program on faculty sensitivity, student success rates, and so on, but you cannot, because you do not have a big enough sample to test hypotheses and you also do not have a comparison group that did not receive the program. You may be able to show that faculty feel more sensitive and students think faculty are more sensitive, and you can show how many students enroll in the program and succeed in completing it, as well as how many plan to practice in a rural area, and so forth. It may be useful to collect qualitative data through interviews with faculty and students to obtain more in-depth data on changes observed and to identify barriers to and facilitators of success in the program.

ORGANIZATIONAL CAPACITY

It is essential to provide reviewers information about your institution so that they can decide whether you are capable of carrying out the program you are proposing. Most proposals include this information after the narrative description of need, target population, and the proposed program and its evaluation. Sometimes proposal writers put the information about their organization right after the introduction, before going into details about the need for the training and the proposed program itself. If you do that, make sure that you have given enough of an overview of the need and your plans to meet the need in the introduction so that readers will not be wondering what this is all about.

Organizational capacity includes several different types of information. The first is the capabilities of the applicant organization. If this is a proposal for a nursing program, what is your nursing school's history? Is it accredited and, if so, by whom? What are its current programs? What is your current enrollment? Graduation rate? What kinds of educational facilities and resources do you have for meeting the needs of those who enroll in the program? Will you do online courses? If so, do you have a system for teaching those? What kind of support do you have from your clinical agencies for adding the new students? If you are in a pharmacy school, social work school, or other health professional school (or college), provide the same kind of information.

The key is to give an overall description of the organization and then describe the organization's abilities to meet the needs of the students you will enroll. For example, it is well known that if you enroll students from a rural area and make them come to the city, they are less likely to go back than if you find a way to train them at home. Thus, if you are focusing on training providers for rural, underserved areas, tell reviewers what resources you have to enable them to get the training they need where they are. If you plan to offer online courses, indicate what technological support you will provide students, and say whether you will do Skyping and use discussion boards and other technologies. Will you use these to help students feel a part of the program? Be sure to indicate the variety of ways you will address the challenges of online education. You may plan to provide online access to journals and other materials through the university library, or you may have support from an Area Health Education Center program or other statewide organization with resources such as libraries. Make these arrangements clear. Perhaps you plan occasional travel by faculty to the area to offer group instruction at a designated meeting place. And if you have developed partnerships with agencies in their area that will provide clinical experiences, indicate that you plan to go to the area at least once or twice a semester to meet one-on-one with students and their preceptors. If faculty plan to provide group instruction, perhaps they can hold these meetings at the same time. Describe these plans in detail. If your proposed program will require any connection to the community, you need to document your linkages with the community and the community support for the proposed work. It is important to include letters of support from any institutions or community groups that will serve as sites or with whom you will be working.

The information in your school's most recent self-study report for accreditation is often very useful for describing organizational capacity. Take a look at the executive summary to see what the document includes and then use the relevant data. You may need to update it, but that's easier than starting from scratch. Do not, however, talk in detail about capacities that are irrelevant. For example, if you do not plan to teach any courses online, do not tell readers about your resources for teaching those courses. If you are not focusing on rural areas, do not talk about linkages to rural organizations—even though your school may have them. Sometimes people writing proposals simply lift the school's or university's boiler plate information about resources and capacities and insert this in the proposal without thinking about what is relevant and what is not. Reviewers will see whether or not you have been thinking about what you need.

It is also important to tell reviewers about the faculty who will direct the program and those who will teach in the program. If you are planning an interprofessional education program, who will be the director? Do you have a team who will administer the program? Have all the departments of those involved agreed to the program? Who will teach what courses? What are their qualifications? Do your faculty have experience in interprofessional teaching? Or practice? It is helpful to give a general description of faculty experience and expertise here, then attach more details, either in biosketches or a table. Will you need to recruit new faculty to teach in the program you are proposing? If so, describe the kinds of faculty you need and the ways you will recruit them. Will you have consultants who are recognized experts in particular areas you are addressing? If so, list them, describe their expertise, and if they have agreed to consult with you, attach letters indicating that.

Once you have shown reviewers the capability of the organization and the faculty to carry out this program, tell them about larger institutional resources. Here again, you can look at the latest self-study report to garner useful information; that information is often found in the introduction to the document but may also be found in the section on resources and facilities available to the school. Think about what you will need to conduct the program—will you need new equipment? Offices? A simulation laboratory? Or access to your school's laboratory? Access to library facilities and services? Do you have all of those? If you are going to be using any technology, it is particularly important to show what kind of technological support will be available to the program. And that information needs to be up to date, not last year's approach.

DETAILED WORK PLAN

This is a monster table (see Table 9.1), and it is often laid out sideways on the paper to make room for all the headings without having long rows of truncated descriptions underneath them. You can also do the table by objective,

TABLE 9.1 Detailed Work Plan for Educational Proposals—Two Options

Objectives	Activities	Timeline	Person(s) Responsible	Outcomes	Evaluation and Benchmarks
Objective 1: (write out in detail) Sub-objective 1.1: (write out in detail) Sub-objective 1.2: (write out in detail) Sub-objective 1.3: (write out in detail)					
Objective 2: (write out in detail) Sub-objective 2.1: (write out in detail) Sub-objective 2.2: (write out in detail) Sub-objective 2.3: (write out in detail)					
Etc.					

Note: Some people create a work plan for each objective, writing the objective first and then including a work plan table for the sub-objectives. For example, they might have the following types of tables.

Objective 1: (write out in detail)

Sub-objectives	Activities	Timeline	Person(s) Responsible	Outcomes	Evaluation and Benchmarks
Sub-objective 1.1: (write out in detail) Sub-objective 1.2: (write out in detail) Sub-objective 1.3: (write out in detail).	List each activity that will be undertaken to accomplish the sub-objective	Indicate year and month(s) activity will occur	Indicate the person(s) responsible for each activity	Indicate what the outcomes will be for each activity	Specify how you will evaluate the success of each activity

Objective 2: (write out in detail)

Sub-objective 2.1: (write out in detail) Sub-objective 2.2: (write out in detail) Sub-objective 2.3: (write out in detail)	List each activity that will be undertaken to accomplish the sub-objective	Indicate year and month(s) activity will occur	Indicate the person(s) responsible for each activity	Indicate what the outcomes will be for each activity	Specify how you will evaluate the success of each activity

which makes it a little more manageable. The table has columns and rows. The columns all have headings: From left to right, they include Objectives, Activities, Timeline, Person(s) Responsible, Outcomes and, finally, Evaluation (and maybe Benchmarks). The rows give all the information about what you will do under these headings. Your objectives will be in the first column; they are clear, having already been stated. But here, in the column under the heading Objectives, you also provide sub-objectives, or the things you must do to achieve the objectives. To articulate these, think about all the things involved in getting to a particular objective or outcome. For example, if your first objective is to enroll more minorities or students from rural underserved areas in your program, then for sub-objectives, you probably will list particular recruitment strategies such as sessions with potential applicants and preparatory work with them to enable them to successfully enroll. As you develop your plans, all of these sub-objectives will become clearer—and then you want to make sure that they are reflected in your narrative on the program, though not presented there as sub-objectives.

In the column to the right of the sub-objectives you list the things you will do to achieve these sub-objectives. Most training grants are 3-year projects, so you need to say whether those activities will occur in Year 1, Year 2, and/or Year 3. To do this, think about how the project will unfold. For example, in Year 1 if your first sub-objective is to increase enrollment of minorities by X number of students, you might meet with guidance counselors in Y number of high schools with high minority student populations, or hold community forums on becoming a health professional. You might talk individually with students enrolled in the freshmen year at the university about strategies for successfully applying to your program. You might also hold workshops for your faculty to ensure that they are sensitive to the problems of minority students. In Years 2 and 3, you may repeat these recruitment strategies and add others. But in Years 2 and 3 you may need to hold sensitivity workshops only for faculty who are new. Think about everything that needs to be done and make good notes. Then put together the activities with the timeline.

In the next column, indicate who will be responsible for each of the activities you have outlined. You may plan to direct the new program, and thus you will be responsible for some of these activities. But you may plan to delegate many activities to other faculty or to other project personnel. Here you must say who will do what. Next indicate your expected outcomes. And finally, you must indicate in detail how you will evaluate the extent to which you meet each sub-objective, your larger objectives, or your proposed outcomes. For example, if you plan to enroll X number of clinicians from rural areas in your state, give the expected figures on enrollment of these clinicians for each year. If you plan to hold workshops for faculty teaching in the program, give expected outcomes—attendance, learning, application in practice.

SUSTAINABILITY AND REPLICABILITY

The training grant is designed to help you start a program—not fund you forever. So it is very important to talk about how you will sustain the program after the funding ends—usually in 3 years. If you do not provide this information, you are not likely to get funded. First off, what will the school do to take this over? It is important to talk to your department chair or your dean and maybe other deans and department chairs, to find out what the school or university is willing to pay for—before you submit the grant proposal, so you can say that we will continue the program after funding ends, based on X. You may need to talk to the person who handles grant budgets and maybe the school's budget officer to figure out how to incorporate this program into the regular curriculum, what the cost will be, and how the school can handle that cost. One way that schools show sustainability is by decreasing the amount of money requested over the years of the grant—can you do that? If so, great. If not, why not? You need to explain. It is not helpful to say that we will seek funding from foundations and other agencies to support the program after the grant funding ends. Either you can take it over or you cannot. Hope does not work, so find the alternative funding before you submit.

In addition to sustaining the program after funding ends, if the program is found useful, it is important to show how you will make it available to others so that they can replicate it. It is helpful to present the program at conferences and through publications, and you should indicate where you plan to present your outcomes and how many publications you expect to complete. But that is not enough. You need to present outcomes to the target population and to the larger community. It is also important to say that you will make the program materials available to those who ask for them and give an email address for that. It is also helpful to say that you will consult on the program with others to help them replicate it.

STATUTORY FUNDING PREFERENCE

Funding preference is given to some applicants based on the following: The project will substantially benefit rural populations or underserved populations or help meet public health needs in state or local health departments. If you receive this preference, you will have a competitive edge over other applicants who are fundable. You must note that you are requesting this preference and document your eligibility for it. For example, if you are applying for funding preference based on your program's potential for serving the underserved, you must explain why you should get this preferred status. Your state or the region of the state you will focus on may be designated by HRSA as an underserved area, and many of the students you enroll may be members of minority and underserved groups. Provide that information—say how many current students and how many prospective students are from underserved areas and populations. Also note whether students will gain information on health indices of these groups and have practical experiences with the underserved populations. It is particularly helpful to partner with schools in historically Black colleges and universities, tribal colleges and universities and institutions serving Hispanics. Also, you want to show that a high rate of graduates work in sites serving underserved populations, and point out the likelihood that your program will improve access and care for the underserved, and continue improving care for the underserved.

MEETING THE REVIEW CRITERIA

At HRSA, your proposal will be reviewed by three persons who are experts in the area. They will use the review criteria that we listed at the beginning of this chapter (as we noted earlier, particular calls may include additional criteria). Each of the reviewers will assess your proposal independently, summarize the review and give the proposal a score from 0 to 100, using the points suggested for each criterion. For example, Response to Program Purpose, which includes the work plan, methods, and resolution of challenges, is worth 30 points—clearly it is extremely important to meet this criterion fully. Then the reviewers will meet in person, by phone, or email to discuss their reviews and come to a consensus on the score. Finally, they will rank the proposal.

The competition for HRSA grants is intense. You want your proposal to get a score as close to 100 as possible so that you have a great chance at getting the money. Therefore, after you have written a draft, go back through the proposal and assess every part of it based on the review criteria; if you see weaknesses, get rid of them or explain them so that they will not be seen as weaknesses. Then have someone else read the proposal with the criteria in mind. If you have time to get comments from an external reviewer, particularly someone who has served as a HRSA reviewer, that will be very helpful. But you have to have time to deal with comments and still submit the proposal on time, so it is useful to make arrangements for a review early in the process. Finally, check everything one last time and send it off. But make sure there are no errors in the sending process!

SECTION III: ADDITIONAL MATERIALS

TEN

TITLE AND ABSTRACT

CREATING A COHERENT TITLE

All proposals need titles. The goal of the title is to tell the reader what the project is about. It should be descriptive and straightforward. If you ramble on forever, you will repeat what is in the text. If it is too short or just sexy, you may not give the reader enough information about the project.

Titles for Research Proposals

In creating a research proposal title, consider the following elements:

- The problem you are studying
- Your focus within the broader problem
- The new approach you have to the problem
- Your focus on a special population, if relevant

Use these elements to craft a title that describes what you propose to do. For example, if you are studying chronic osteoarthritis, what are you focusing on within this topic area? What is the exact problem that you are addressing? Are you intervening to produce a certain result? Are you focusing on a special group that is in particular need? Use your answers to these questions to create versions of your title. For example:

- The problem is pain
- In particular, you might wish to reduce knee pain

- Using a new intervention that involves gentle exercise
- In older adults with chronic osteoarthritis

You might start with a title like this:

> *Reducing Knee Pain in Older Adults With Chronic Osteoarthritis (62 characters and spaces)*

But while this title has many of the needed elements, it is lacking the mention of the new approach to solving knee pain in this population. So, without deleting the original title, elaborate it:

> *Intervening Using Gentle Exercise to Reduce Knee Pain in Older Adults With Chronic Osteoarthritis (97 characters and spaces)*

This title is too long for many agencies. For example, in the recent past, the National Institutes of Health (NIH) only allowed a total of 81 characters including spaces for a title (it does sound short, but in even older days, NIH only allowed 56 characters including spaces!). To achieve this, get rid of the unnecessary words in the title:

> *Gentle Exercise to Reduce Knee Pain in Older Adults With Chronic Osteoarthritis (79 characters and spaces)*

It is easiest to do this using a convenient software program such as Microsoft Word:

1. List the elements that should be in your title.
2. Craft a title.
3. Use "word count" in "review" to count the number of characters including spaces; type this number after the title.
4. Then, without deleting anything, begin fiddling with the title—does it need to be shorter? Did you leave out something crucial? Remember to keep all your versions of the title with their character/space counts so you can cull from them what you might wish to try in another version.
5. Get feedback from others about your title; revise as needed.

The NIH has now changed most of its applications to allow longer title lengths. Two hundred characters including spaces are now allowed for research grants, fellowships, and career development awards. This length matches what some other agencies allow, but we encourage you to be succinct and not to use all 200 characters and spaces unless you really need to (you might want to consider something like the American Psychological Association's [APA] maximum allowed length of 12 words for journal article titles). It is hard to get your message across with a really long title—it gives you a lot of room in which to be wishy-washy and does not necessarily require you to think hard about what you are hoping to do. It is a godsend, however, if you need a few extra characters to finish your title.

A few "don'ts": Don't oversell—don't say you are curing cancer if you are not. You don't want readers to be disappointed once they read your proposal. Don't use language that differs from the language you use in the text, even if it is shorter. A classic example of this is using "Black" in the title and "African American" in the text—be consistent! Don't use special characters unless you are sure they will work in the application packet you use to submit the proposal. And whatever you do, don't use more characters and spaces than the guidelines allow. While publishers might work with your title, the NIH typically just lops your title off in the middle of a word, so it is better to keep it within the guidelines. Examples of the "lop off" might include endings like "... Pain Management in Ch" and "... Using." The reader doesn't know what "Ch" means, and "Using" what? Remember that these truncated titles stay with you for years, even appearing in the NIH electronic records that the entire world can see via the NIH's website.

Titles for Educational Training Grant Proposals

Most educational training grant proposals follow very similar guidelines to those outlined for research titles. You have chosen the program because there is a need, but you will describe that need in the text not in the title. So in your title include:

1. What the program is
2. Whom it is for

For HRSA grants, for example, there may be layers of titles related to the program to which you are applying, followed by your particular title. Your proposal might be targeted for geriatric education centers, workforce diversity, advanced education, interprofessional collaborative practice, or other programs. You can move on from these programmatic titles and assume that they are known when titling your proposal. Within the overall program to which you are applying, what is your program and whom is it for? Be specific. Are you proposing to prepare family nurse practitioners? In anything in particular? For example, will your program teach them about caring for children with chronic conditions? Then you might have a title like this:

Preparing Family Nurse Practitioners to Care for Children With Chronic Conditions

Perhaps, you wish to add coursework and experience to the preparation of graduate students that will enhance their ability to collaborate with other providers when they are caring for children with chronic conditions. You might have a title like this:

Training Health-Provider Graduate Students to Work Collaboratively When Dealing With Children With Chronic Conditions

Follow the guidelines provided previously for research titles: (a) List the elements that you believe should be in your title; (b) craft a title; (c) if the program to which you are applying has a limit on the number of characters (and perhaps spaces), use "word count" in your software program to count them and type this number after the title; (d) if needed, fiddle with the title to make it clearer and keep it within the space guidelines; and (e) get feedback from others and revise as needed.

Some people include acronyms in their titles; other people do not. It is your call. The only rule is to make sure that the title is clear: If the title creates an acronym, put it in parentheses at the end of the title; if you are using an acronym as part of the title, use it as desired in the title but make sure it is spelled out early in the text so the reader is not left wondering about it for too long!

WRITING AN EFFECTIVE ABSTRACT

The abstract is one of the most important parts of any proposal you write—because all reviewers pay close attention to it. Abstracts for proposals to the NIH are especially important because not all reviewers read the full proposal carefully: They may have to read as many as 60 or 70 proposals and critique several of those, so they do not have time to look at everything in the proposals they are not critiquing. However, they all read the abstract, relying on it to give them a quick understanding of the study and its potential impact. Your task is to provide that understanding in 30 lines or fewer, not a word over. Other agencies may allow more space, but they all have limits, so read the guidelines carefully and never go over those limits. Reviewers for those agencies may also be reviewing numerous proposals, so here too an informative abstract is essential.

Writing a good abstract is not easy, but it is doable with some effort. First of all, never write the abstract until you are close to having a final draft of the proposal or you will have to rewrite it countless times as your ideas change. But do not wait until the last minute and slap something together, or you will have a terribly disjointed product and that will reduce your chances of getting funded. Plan to write several drafts of the abstract, just as you do for the proposal.

An abstract needs to tell readers quickly why a study is needed, what its purpose is, who will be studied, what the intervention is (if there is one), what data will be collected, and how the data will be analyzed. Never write the first draft to space specifications, or you will leave out half the essentials. Write what you think needs to be included and then cut back later as you are refining.

The most difficult part of writing the abstract (as with the proposal) is making the case for the study—showing the need and concisely stating the purpose. In NIH proposals, the rationale for the study and its purpose are generally stated in the opening two paragraphs of the Specific Aims section. Pick those up and use them to begin. Look also at what you have written about need in your Significance section and make sure you have the right emphasis. For example, if you are interested in reducing the prevalence of hepatitis C in a particular population group, you have probably talked at length in the Significance section about the evidence documenting the prevalence in this group and showing that efforts to reduce the prevalence have not had major effect—which is why you plan to try a new approach. You may have said that more quickly in Specific Aims. Look at both and condense the information into two sentences: "Hepatitis C is a particular problem in Group X, with a prevalence of Y, but no interventions to date have successfully reduced the prevalence. Therefore, we plan to test the effectiveness of a new strategy, Z, for preventing infection in this group." These two sentences give both the rationale for the study and its purpose.

If your proposal is going to an agency or organization other than the NIH, look at your introductory or background material to find what you have said about the need for the study; usually you will find that information just before the study purpose. Do not, however, say something vague such as: "There is a gap in the literature on X." That sentence does not tell readers anything about what the problem is or what needs to be done about it. And remember—not every gap needs to be filled. (And if you have used a sentence like that in the body of the proposal, rewrite it to be more specific.) You need to clearly articulate the particular problem or part of a problem that you plan to address, and then give the purpose. And that purpose is never to "fill a gap in the literature"; the purpose is always something specific.

If you are planning to examine the factors affecting a problem or to test an intervention, you probably will also have some specific aims. For example, if you plan to try a new approach to preventing HIV infection in a hard-to-reach group, you may intend to test the effectiveness of (a) community involvement, (b) outreach efforts, and (c) immediate feedback on testing. When you draft the abstract, include these specific aims, recognizing that later you may have to drop them because of space problems.

Most research proposals also include hypotheses or research questions. Often, however, these overlap with the specific aims, and therefore you can save space by deleting one or the other. For example, if your aims are to examine the efficacy of an intervention in altering adolescent views of the acceptability of violence and reducing adolescent perpetration of violence, you do not need to tell reviewers all that and then say that you hypothesize that adolescents who receive the intervention will view violence as less acceptable and in turn carry out less violence than a control group. Look at the aims and hypotheses or questions and decide which version gives the most information about the study in the fewest words. In this case, you may want to skip aims and give the hypotheses.

After stating purpose and aims (hypotheses and/or questions), move to approach or methods. Do not include preliminary work unless it is absolutely crucial to your plans. If reviewers need to know about preliminary work in order to understand the reasoning behind your methods, you have to provide that information in one sentence. (Don't, however, refer reviewers to a later section that describes preliminary work; the abstract needs to be self-contained.)

Remember that reviewers who only skim the proposal will not gain any information on study methods unless you provide it here. To give a succinct description of methods, look at the opening sentences of your Methods section, on the study design. Use that overview and elaborate as much as space will allow, including participants, intervention (if there is one), and data to be collected. First tell readers who you will study; for example, you might say "The study will recruit 120 African American men who are prehypertensive, 60 for the intervention and 60 for the control group." Next, describe the intervention or program, if you are testing one. This also needs to be said quickly. For example, if you are planning to implement a 10-session family intervention to help African American women better manage their weight and prevent weight gain in their children, you do not have room to say much about it here. You must say in a sentence or at most two sentences, what the intervention will involve. For example, "A 10-session intervention will engage mothers and children in complementary education and coping skills classes and joint sessions on cooking and exercising." Look at the introductory sentences in your description of the intervention in the proposal; often they give the essence and you can just copy them.

Then you must tell the readers what data you will collect. Writers often fail to indicate how they will measure study variables, but this information is essential. Otherwise reviewers have no idea how you will test the efficacy of an intervention or answer questions about the issue being studied. Look at the section on variables and their measurement in the proposal and if you have written one or two sentences to introduce that section, use those sentences for the abstract. If you have not provided an introduction to your section on variables and their measurement, pull out the main sentences in this section. For example, if you plan to collect data on biomarkers, say in one sentence what data on which biomarkers you will collect, but do not give the details. If you plan to use instrument X to collect data on depression, and instrument Y to collect data on anxiety, you may want to say that, but you do not always need to give the names of instruments; you can simply say that you will collect data on depression and anxiety—that's what's important. Use your judgment about whether you need to name the instrument. If you do list instruments, do not use acronyms or abbreviations; give the full titles of the instruments. Finally, if you are examining the feasibility of an intervention, you will probably collect data to determine whether implementation of the treatment is successful: Don't forget to include the measures you will use to evaluate success (recruitment? retention? acceptance? utility?).

The abstract must also indicate how the data will be analyzed. This needs to be succinct, so do not repeat the entire data analysis section of your proposal. Focus on the main aims of the study. For example, "To evaluate the efficacy of the intervention, we will use multivariate analyses of co-variance and multinomial logistic regression techniques." Unless you have an analysis-focused or -intensive study, this is probably all you need in the abstract.

Finally, it is also helpful to give one concluding sentence about the potential impact of the study. For example, if you are testing a new approach to diabetes management, you might conclude thus: "If this intervention is found efficacious, it may provide a model for diabetes management and a model for management of other chronic diseases."

After you have written a draft of the abstract, print it double spaced, count the words and lines, look at what you have written, and begin revising. First make sure that you have covered everything that needs to be said. Does the abstract show the need for the study; are the purpose and aims clear; does it look like the study can be carried out with the methods you propose; is there reason to think the findings will have an impact on the science and on practice; and is the material presented in a logical order? If you are not sure whether you have included all the essential information, it may be helpful to look at other people's abstracts. A colleague may have a proposal abstract that you can look at. If there is no one in your university or agency who has a proposal that you can look at, try looking at abstracts written in published articles. Everything up to the Findings will be useful in helping you see what is essential. You can also check the NIH Reporter for abstracts. You will find it under the Grants and Funding link on the NIH website.

Once you have presented all the essential information, your abstract will probably be twice as long as it should be—more like 60 lines than 30 lines. Before you start cutting, however, it is helpful to have someone else read the abstract and tell you whether it makes sense. Then, if your reader finds holes in the logic or sentences that do not seem relevant, revise to make the abstract coherent.

Once you are convinced that the draft is complete and logical, start cutting back. First, look at redundancies; often you can cut whole sentences because you have made a point twice using only slightly different words. Next, look at information that may be interesting but is not essential. This kind of extra information is often found in the description of the need for the study and in the description of the intervention you are testing. Cut back. Each time you cut, print the abstract again, check the number of lines, and read the abstract again for logic and clarity. And finally, start cutting out words. There are many "the's" that can be dropped, and long words can often be replaced by shorter words. For example, "physician" can be replaced by "doctor" or "MD"; you should say "use," not "utilize," and most "withins" are really "ins." Cut until you are at 30 lines for the NIH or whatever the agency you are going to requires. Then read once more to be sure you have said everything essential and it is clear and in the right order. And always go back one last time before you submit the proposal, to be sure that you are consistent with the last proposal draft. You do not want to say in your abstract that your study will include 150 people when you have realized that you can only afford 75 and have made that change in the body of the proposal.

WRITING THE PROJECT NARRATIVE

For NIH proposals, applicants are required to provide a "project narrative" in addition to the abstract. The project narrative is short—the NIH requests two to three sentences that describe the importance of the research to public health. Write it in lay language that can be understood by a broad audience. This is what is used to tell Congress about the research that NIH is funding. Think "elevator speech": brief and to the point. It is best to write this narrative after you have a final draft of the abstract. Otherwise you will say too much, and you are likely to give the wrong emphasis. When your abstract is clear, this is easier to do. Look at your sentences on need and purpose and your concluding sentence on the potential impact of the study, and condense those to a couple of clear sentences about the importance of your work.

ELEVEN

BIOGRAPHICAL INFORMATION

When you are writing a proposal for someone who knows you (e.g., a PhD proposal or a Doctor of Nursing Practice [DNP] proposal), you typically are not required to provide extra information about who you are. The folks know you, so the information is redundant. However, when you are writing a proposal to be sent to a foundation, an agency, and sometimes even your own institution, you are often required to tell people about yourself, and when appropriate, your team members. Why? Because the reviewers probably don't know you and want information with which to evaluate you. Some of that determination is made based on the quality of what you have written in the proposal, but reviewers often also want to know where you were educated, what sorts of positions you have held, whether you have had other funding, and whether you have published your findings. How do you provide all of this information? All proposal programs will tell you exactly what they want, but it is usually some shortened form of your curriculum vitae (CV).

NATIONAL INSTITUTES OF HEALTH (NIH) BIOSKETCH INFORMATION

The NIH uses what is called a "biosketch," which is just a short form of your CV with some restrictions (e.g., biosketches are limited in the number of pages allowed—currently five). Why these restrictions? Because people like to go on and on and on about how wonderful they are, and senior people have *very* long CVs because they have been in the business a long time. The NIH is interested only in the most salient information; hence, the restrictions. As noted later, the NIH has different rules for the biosketches for different types of grants.

Biosketch for Research Grant Proposals

Most NIH research grant applications and many other agencies use the traditional (general) NIH biosketch as a format to request information about you, your team members, and other key personnel. The NIH website has both a blank biosketch form and a completed sample form to guide you in its use. (These can be accessed in the Biosketches section after you click on the SF424 [R&R] to access the application guidelines. Remember that you want to match the version to what you chose for the SF424 [R&R], which these days is version C. Also, you can now build your biosketch using Science Experts Network Curriculum Vitae [SciENcv] if you wish.)

A lot of the information required at the beginning is easy to figure out because it has rather obvious labels, but even here there are questions. For example, is "name" presented last name first or first name first? Either format is acceptable, but it would be good to present all the names in a consistent format in your application. What about "position title"? People tend to put a lot of information here that is not really needed; all the NIH really wants is your current position title at your institution. This is not your position title if you get the grant, or your position title if you hope to get tenure before the grant is funded and so on—it is your current position title. If you are an assistant professor? Say so. If you are an associate professor? Say so. This is very simple unless you hold lots of positions at the primary institution and need to name them all (in which case, just list them!).

The electronic Research Administration Commons (eRA Commons) User Name probably needs a bit of explanation. The eRA Commons is how the NIH communicates with people who apply for grants, and it is where you can follow your grant through the system and get your score and reviews. Therefore, all principal investigators (PIs) are required to sign up to participate in the eRA Commons, be assigned a name, and create a password *before* they submit their grants. Usually, the NIH has approved someone at your institution to sign people up for the eRA Commons, so ask the research administration folks in your department or institution who can help you. The NIH wants you to put the name you are assigned (not the password!) on the biosketch so they know how to contact you. Your team members may also have eRA Commons names, and those can be entered on their respective biosketches, but as of now, the eRA Commons name is only required for PIs (and primary sponsors of National Research Service Awards [NRSAs]).

The next section of the biosketch is a table where you list your education and formal training. Beginning with your baccalaureate or other initial professional degree, list all your degrees, certifications, and formal postdoctoral training in chronological order. All you have to do is read the instructions on the form and follow them; it is not rocket science. But many, many people either don't put the information in chronological order (from oldest to newest) or don't put the location of the institution or leave something else out. Don't be one of those people.

After the education table you put "**A. Personal Statement.**" This section is usually one to two paragraphs that briefly describe the experience and qualifications that make you particularly well suited for your role on the proposed project. What you cover may overlap with the studies you write about in the preliminary work section, but the personal statement allows you more latitude in describing your role in the proposed study, skills you learned, perhaps how you became interested in the topic area, and so on. This is also where you have the opportunity to talk about things in your life that might have affected your scientific advancement or productivity. Perhaps you took time out to raise children or care for a family member; talk about these things and the impact they have had on your progress as a researcher, but remember that the reader should be left with a positive impression about you and what you can contribute to the proposed project. The NIH allows you to list up to four relevant publications at the end of this section that highlight your experience and qualifications. Just make sure that you don't list the same publications in Section C.

Hopefully, all of your team members will have adapted the personal statements they have written for themselves to be appropriate for their roles on this particular project. If they haven't? Don't just include each biosketch as it is given to you. Once you have reviewed it, if changes need to be made, either ask the person to adapt it, explaining why and perhaps giving some guidance to make it fit your project, or ask the person whether you can adapt it as long as you send the adaptation to the person for final approval (and be sure to seek that approval!).

The next section is: "**B. Positions and Honors.**" Most investigators break this into sections, using the same format for all of them. For example, a person might use three sections: Positions and Employment, Other Experience and Professional Memberships, and Honors and Awards. Under each, list the year or range of years applicable to the item on the left and then tab over and provide the details on that particular item. Put items in chronological order, using the date when you started in a position, professional membership, and so on. If, for example, you started a membership in 2002 and it goes through the present, you would put it before something that started in 2004, no matter when the membership ended (even if it is still going on). By the way, the NIH asks you to be sure to include current memberships on any federal government public advisory committees.

In the next section, "**C. Contributions to Science,**" the NIH asks you to briefly describe up to five of your most significant contributions to science. For each contribution, include a brief paragraph about the scientific contribution you have made, its impact, and up to four publications and non-publication research products. Don't duplicate anything you listed in the Personal Statement and include public access information (e.g., PubMed Central identification numbers) where you can. You have up to half a page for each contribution, but just be sure to stay within the overall five-page limit for the biosketch.

The NIH allows any reference format as long as it is complete and used consistently; for nursing, the American Psychological Association (APA) style is generally preferred, but not required. Different people interpret the word "consistently" differently: Some think it means within each biosketch while others think all biosketches in one proposal should use the same reference format. We will leave this interpretation to you, but making them all consistent does take time and expertise! Remember also, for anyone who has had a name change within their references, it is helpful to add some sort of note so the reader can understand what has happened—it can be confusing if you do not know that "Smith" and "Jones" are the same person. In this section, the NIH also allows you to include a URL to a full list of your publications in a publicly available database, such as My Bibliography or SciENcv—both of which are available via the National Library of Medicine (NLM). The NIH biosketch webpage and forms found there give you the links to these resources.

The last section of a biosketch is "D. Research Support." Please note that this is *not* the same thing as "other support," which is not submitted with the proposal. Research Support includes current research funding as well as what the person has had for the past 3 years. When completing a biosketch, include any type of research support you have had—not just federal funding. Include both foundation funding and competitive institutional research awards (although monies for which you did not compete, such as start-up funds, usually are not included here). The sample biosketch page referred to previously gives an excellent format for including this information, but do include the grant number (if there is one), the PI's name, the dates of the award, the project title, a brief description of the project (one to two sentences maximum), and your role on the project. Sometimes there is overlap (e.g., if you are the named PI, is it not clear that your role is as PI?); use your best judgment to decide whether to include both bits of information or whether to delete the latter one because it is not needed. When in doubt, use both!

Biosketch for Career Development Award (K) Proposals

If you are submitting a Career Development Award application (perhaps for a K01 or K23), your mentor(s) should use the biosketch format outlined previously. However, for you, there are a few differences. Use the same form, but in the Personal Statement your goal is to explain why your experience and qualifications make you particularly well suited to receive the award for which you are applying. Instead of the Positions and Honors section, you are asked to use the heading Research and/ or Professional Experience. Under that heading you should have three subcategories: Employment, Honors, and Professional Societies and Public Advisory Committees. In the Employment category, you are asked to provide all of your employment positions since receiving your baccalaureate, from oldest to newest. A small table is usually recommended in which, for each position, you include department or organization, department head or supervisor, rank, tenured if applicable, full or part time, and inclusive dates (month and year). Yikes! This means that you have to have fairly complete records, so be sure to keep an accounting of such details if you think you will apply for a K award in the future. Under its own subheading, Honors should be listed chronologically. Include both academic and professional honors, as well as research grants and competitive fellowships. (Yes, this latter category might overlap with the Research Support section, but you can just add a note about the overlap to make it clear that you are not trying to "double dip.") Next, list Professional Societies and Public Advisory Committees for the past 10 years.

The last two sections, Contributions to Science and Research Support, are the same as for the traditional biosketch.

Biosketch for Fellowship Proposals

The fellowship biosketch forms and completed samples can be found after the traditional general biosketch in the Biosketch section (after you click on SF424 [R&R] to access the application guidelines). You will notice that there are some differences in the fellowship biosketch instructions, although much of the format is identical to the traditional biosketch format. First and foremost, because these fellowships are for pre- and postdoctoral applicants, the reviewers won't expect you to have the same level of scientific productivity as a more senior investigator. And as you are not likely to be very far along in your scientific career, things such as course work and your performance in courses matter. As with the traditional biosketch, you are allowed up to five pages for your presentation of the information.

The first place you will probably see a difference is in the Personal Statement. You should use this statement to show why your experience and qualifications make you particularly well suited for the fellowship. This will probably take one to two paragraphs and overlap a bit with other training sections. Be sure to include the most relevant of your experiences, your long-term goals, and what the training and research experience you propose in the fellowship will enable you to accomplish in the area of research. Remember that the NIH pre- and postdoctoral fellowships are training you to be a researcher—not a teacher or a clinician—so keep the focus on research.

As is true for those completing the traditional NIH biosketch, up to four publications may be included in this section to highlight your experience and qualifications. (Note the additional instructions in this section for applicants for certain awards.)

In the Positions and Honors section, the NIH provides a table for you to complete for all non-degree training and employment. In the table, they ask you to list the activity or occupation, beginning and ending dates, field, institution or company, and supervisor or employer. Yes, it is a lot of information, so hopefully you have kept good records. After this table, list any Academic and Professional Honors, including scholarships, traineeships, fellowships, development awards, poster awards, and so on, along with their respective dates, titles, and locations. Membership in Professional Societies is next. This should include current memberships in such societies, along with the date or date range, role you have in the organization, and society name. At this point in your career, the "role" is probably "member," but as you progress in your career, you will want to seek contributing roles and leadership in relevant organizations.

The Contributions to Science section is also done a bit differently from the traditional biosketch. Although you are allowed to describe up to five contributions, pre- and postdoctoral applicants are encouraged to consider highlighting only two or three that they consider to be most important. As with the traditional biosketch, up to four publications can be listed for each contribution, but applicants are encouraged to group the publications for each contribution into categories (research papers, abstracts, book chapters, and reviews), putting items in each grouping in chronological order (from oldest to newest). As with the traditional biosketch, no particular reference format is required, but whatever you choose should be complete and consistent, and public access information should be included when available (e.g., URLs, PubMed Central IDs). You are also allowed to include manuscripts pending publication or even in preparation, and a URL that links to a listing of all of your published work is allowed. Be sure to note any name changes you have had that appear in your publications.

A Scholastic Performance section is next. Predoctoral applicants are asked to give a complete list of all undergraduate and graduate courses with grades in the chart provided. If you have attended multiple schools, try to organize the information by semester so it makes logical sense to the reviewer. If the grading system for any of the courses differs from the standard A to F, explain the system so it can be understood by reviewers. At the time of application, you are not asked to provide transcripts, although they may be requested down the line, so you might want to go ahead and request official copies just in case.

Postdoctoral applicants provide information on scholastic performance as well, but they do not have to provide the information for all courses. They are asked to list, by institution and year, undergraduate and graduate scientific and/or professional courses germane to the training sought under the award. Grades are also to be provided, and nonstandard grading systems must be explained.

The fellowship biosketches do not request the Research Support section required on the traditional biosketch. Why? Well, the NIH knows that you are earlier in your research career and are more likely to have had the type of support that is requested in the Academic and Professional Honors section. If you have grant support, feel free to put it in that section as well.

Just as you do with the proposal text, get your primary sponsor to review the biosketch and provide input. Make sure that your sponsor reads the personal statement with an eye toward making sure it reads well and makes a coherent argument about why you are ideal for the fellowship. Also, if there are any shortcomings in your past performance that appear on the biosketch (perhaps low grades early in your academic career?), the sponsor should address the issue in the Sponsor section. Thus, you do not need to explain the situation on the biosketch; the Sponsor does the explaining in her or his section.

Graduate Board Examination (GRE) scores are no longer requested, even for predoctoral fellowship applicants! For the traditional and fellow biosketches, we recommend that applicants keep a close eye on changes in the guidelines so that they use whatever guidance is appropriate for their application deadline.

BIOGRAPHICAL INFORMATION FOR NON-NIH PROPOSALS

What if you are submitting an application to an agency other than the NIH—what will be expected for the biosketches? While different agencies or foundations may request a different format or page length, many either use the NIH biosketch form or allow you to substitute the NIH form for theirs. However, whether they allow an identical form or not, you will be well served by the content listed earlier for the NIH—these are the types of information that are requested for many types of research grant applications (e.g., American Cancer Society, American Nurses Foundation, Robert Wood Johnson Foundation, Sigma Theta Tau International).

If you are writing a proposal for an educational project, for example, via Health Resources and Services Administration (HRSA), it also accepts the NIH biosketch, but as biosketches count in the page limits for HRSA, you will want to reduce them to as few pages as possible—perhaps even one page for each person except the project director, for whom you might wish to allow two pages (if needed). As research funding is less critical, you will want to remove that section of the biosketch, and most people also remove the personal statement due to space limitations. You will want to scrunch everything else down, perhaps including only the most relevant few publications (although you might want to include a summary statement such as "Peer-reviewed publications selected from over 40 books, articles, and chapters") so the reviewer knows that you have actively published. Clearly, though, if you have lots and lots of people on your proposal, you will take up many of the allowed pages with biosketches, so be judicious in whom you ask to be a member of your project team.

TWELVE

BUDGET

INTRODUCTION

Why in heaven would you want to learn how to develop a budget for a proposal when you have folks who can help you with the process and you need to focus your efforts on writing the proposal and designing the project?

The answer is easy: Unless you, the principal investigator or program director, are involved in the budgeting process, you would not know (a) whether you can perform all of the activities with the money requested, or (b) whether the distribution of funds over budget periods is appropriate for your project. The work you are proposing should drive the budget.

How do you go about creating the budget yourself or guiding the person who might be helping you?

- First and foremost, you *must* know the budget guidelines of the funder/funding program. What sorts of costs do they allow? What is the maximum budget you may have in any one year? Is there a cap on salaries? Is overhead (also called indirects or, in the federal government's parlance, facilities and administration [F&A]) allowed, and is it "in" the cap allowed by the funding opportunity or "in addition" to it? Thus, read the funding opportunity announcement (FOA) closely—for the federal government, you will typically find FOAs on the www.grants.gov website; in addition, the National Institutes of Health (NIH) lists its FOAs in the NIH Guide for Grants and Contracts on its website; and foundations list their FOAs on their own websites as well as on summary sites such as The Foundation Center (see Chapter 1). Most institutions have negotiated F&A rates with the federal government and only allow lesser amounts for certain grants when the cap on the F&A rate is clearly specified in writing (e.g., for fellowships, training grants, career development awards, and small research grants).

- Second, you need to know what your approach (design and methods) will be and the timeline for these activities before a budget can be developed. If you are just starting the process, develop your project's aims and at least outline the design and methods, with a timeline, before beginning the budget. You need to know what you are going to do and when in order to estimate how much it will cost.

- Third, remember that your goal is to have an appropriate budget—one that fits within the guidelines of the program to which you are applying and also covers your costs as much as possible. Appropriateness, not size, is the goal.

Research Budget

Think through the approach you will take to your research and all the activities that will be associated with it. Examples (using the NIH budget categories from the SF424 [R&R] which can be found at www.grants.nih. gov/grants/funding/424/index.htm) include:

- **Personnel costs**: Who will be doing what, when will they be doing it, and how long it will take? Think through and list all the activities of the project, and make a timeline for them. Begin with start-up activities such as hiring, training, copying/preparing materials, and informing sites that have agreed to participate; then move on to activities such as recruitment, data collection, intervention, data entry and cleaning, analysis, and report/ article writing. List them all, then indicate who will do each task and how long the task will take for each research subject. You may need several types of people to successfully execute your grant activities (recruiters, data collectors, interventionists, data coders, programmers), or you may be able to combine some of the activities into one position as long as that does not introduce bias into your study. Make sure to specify the time needed each month, so you can estimate the time needed for each person in each fiscal period of the grant. And do not forget travel time! Tally the hours for each type of person so you know how much of their time will be needed. Do this for both the staff you will hire on the grant and for the "key personnel" (investigators), who also have important work to do— overseeing the project; training, monitoring, and retraining staff; analyzing data; writing reports and articles; and so on. It often helps to make separate charts for the investigators and the staff of a project. The charts you make can serve as a guide to the person who is going to help you create the budget. Often, that person can help you determine the salary and fringe-benefit rates for each investigator or staff person (see Table 12.1).

TABLE 12.1 Sample Calculation of Staff Hours Needed to Conduct Study

Design: Two-group experimental design
Intervention: Four monthly intervention visits in the home
Data Collection: At baseline, immediately postintervention, and 3 months following end of intervention
Subject Number: 66 subjects per group
Staff Needed: RA support (for data collection, etc.) and nurse support (for the intervention)

Tasks	Who	Time	Travel	Y1 M1	Y1 M2	Y1 M3	Y1 M4	Y1 M5	Y1 M6	Y1 M7	Y1 M8	Y1 M9	Y1 M10	Y1 M11	Y1 M12	Y2 M1	Y2 M2	Y2 M3	Y2 M4	Y2 M5	Y2 M6	Y2 M7	Y2 M8	Y2 M9	Y2 M10	Y2 M11	Y2 M12	RA Y1 n Ss	RA Y1 hrs/S	RA Y1 tot hrs	RA Y2 n Ss	RA Y2 hrs/S	RA Y2 tot hrs	Nurse Y1 n Ss	Nurse Y1 hrs/S	Nurse Y1 tot hrs	Nurse Y2 n Ss	Nurse Y2 hrs/S	Nurse Y2 tot hrs
Hire RAs	RA	20 hrs		▓	▓	▓																								20									
Train RAs	Nurse	60 hrs		▓	▓	▓																														60			
Train interventionists	Nurse	40 hrs		▓	▓	▓																																	
Prep and copy materials	RA	40 hrs		▓	▓	▓																								40									
Contact sites	Nurse	20 hrs																																		20			
Intervention Subjects																																								
Subject recruitment (n)	RA	2 hrs	at clinic				4	6	8	8	8	8	8	8	8													66	2	132									
Baseline data collection	RA	1 hr	at clinic				4	6	8	8	8	8	8	8	8													66	1	66									
Intervention visit 1	Nurse	2 hrs	50 mi/1 hr					4	6	8	8	8	8	8	8	8																		58	3	174	8	3	24
Intervention visit 2	Nurse	2 hrs	50 mi/1 hr						4	6	8	8	8	8	8	8	8																	50	3	150	16	3	48
Intervention visit 3	Nurse	2 hrs	50 mi/1 hr							4	6	8	8	8	8	8	8	8																42	3	126	24	3	72
Intervention visit 4	Nurse	2 hrs	50 mi/1 hr								4	6	8	8	8	8	8	8	8														34	3	102	32	3	96
Immediate post data collection	RA	1 hr	50 mi/1 hr								4	6	8	8	8	8	8	8	8							34	2	68	32	2	64						
3-month follow-up data collection	RA	1 hr	50 mi/1 hr											4	6	8	8	8	8	8	8	8				10	2	20	56	2	112						
Control Subjects																																								
Subject recruitment (n)	RA	1 hr	at clinic				4	6	8	8	8	8	8	8	8													66	2	132									
Baseline data collection	RA	1 hr	at clinic				4	6	8	8	8	8	8	8	8													66	1	66									
Immediate post data collection	RA	1 hr	50 mi/1 hr								4	6	8	8	8	8	8	8	8							34	2	68	32	2	64						
3-month follow up data collection	RA	1 hr	50 mi/1 hr											4	6	8	8	8	8	8	8	8				10	2	20	56	2	112						
Data Management and Analysis																																								
Data coding and cleaning	RA																																							
Data entry	RA																																							
Data analysis programming	RA																																							
Continue with other tasks as appropriate…																																								
																													632			352			632			240

Data Management and Analysis note: Continue estimating for all tasks … transition to shading boxes instead of inserting subject numbers as appropriate

Numbers in cells are the numbers of subjects

Convert these hour estimates to a percent time and then to "person months" for NIH applications:
1. There are 2080 hours in a full-time workload for 1 year; assume about 80 are vacation; thus divide the total hours needed by 2000 to get a percent time
2. Multiply the percent time by months of the type appointment to get person months

RA, research assistant.

Becauses it is difficult to compare the percentages of time different people will devote to grant activities when they are on different types of appointments (e.g., some faculty are on 9-month appointments, some on 12-month appointments), the NIH asks that all personnel time requests be made in "person months." While most folks find this challenging, it is actually quite easy to calculate: Merely multiply the percentage of time you have determined you need of each person by the months of their appointment. So, 10% of a 12-month appointee, is 1.2 person months. For someone on a 9-month appointment, 10% would be .9 person months if you only need them during the academic year. But if you also need the person during the three summer months, you also specify .3 summer months. It is important to remember that most research is a year-round endeavor, so plan accordingly! (And no, you do not want to show a huge bump-up in percent time/person months during the summer just because you want summer money—the person months you request must match the work to be done.)

The data you enter into Table 12.1 also provide you the data you need to make another important determination: who should be on your grant and in the budget. If a person has nothing to contribute to the grant, that person should not be on it. An NIH grant is not a popularity contest—you only want to include investigators and staff who will give real effort to the endeavor. One exception to this might be people who will contribute their time. Perhaps you are a new investigator and a senior investigator is willing to contribute her or his time to mentor you through the research process. That person should be on the grant. But remember, there is no room for redundancies—it is not cost efficient to have multiple people doing the same thing (and it can be frustrating!).

- **Nonpersonnel costs:**
  - *Equipment*: Most institutions use this category only for equipment that is so expensive it totals more than $5,000 per unit. Remember that unless you are applying for an equipment grant, you will not want to load your budget up with lots of equipment that you will only be using for a short while. Look for ways to share the equipment that people are using on other projects.
  - *Travel:* Usually you will want to consider two types of travel: (a) travel to conduct the study and (b) professional travel to meetings. The former should be estimated carefully for each subject you will have in the study; be sure to count round-trip travel costs for your staff or for the subject. Parking, lodging, and other travel costs need to be estimated for trips for recruitment, data collection, and intervention. The NIH allows professional travel on most grants, but be sure to check the FOA! And remember that for most research projects, you would not have results to present in the early years of

the study, so you may not have professional travel until later in the project period. Moreover, your budget may not be able to accommodate all investigators traveling in all of the data-presentation years. Be frugal!

- *Materials and supplies:* If you are going to include computers, be sure they are well justified and will be necessary for the conduct of the research. Ditto for printers and peripherals, toner, paper, flash drives, and the like. Materials might also include any copying needs; software purchases; recruitment, retention, intervention, and data collection supplies; and audio and video recorders, to name but a few possibilities. Personalize these expenses to the needs of your study.
- *Consultant costs:* Will you have one or more consultants (experts outside your institution)? If so, you will want to include any related costs in the budget. If there will be an hourly or daily fee, include it. Also, costs related to the travel of consultants to your study site should be included here (your travel to see them would be included under "travel"). However, be as frugal as possible. Consider using the consultants only at critical times, and consider using phone, e-mail and Skype in lieu of in-person visits when possible.
- *Computer services*: Will someone or some unit be assisting you with computer setup, maintenance, and repair? If so, include the fees here.
- *Subawards/consortial/contractual costs:* If scholars at another institution or agency will be participating in the science of your project, you may need to set up a formal subcontract with that institution so their expenses can be folded into your budget. This can be a time-consuming process, so start early! Note that, typically, you do not need to create a subcontract for sites that are just providing access to subjects—usually these sites do not have someone who is contributing to the science of the project.
- *Equipment or facility rental/user fees:* Here is where you include any fees associated with using a site, perhaps for providing the intervention to subjects or for collecting their data.
- *Other (1, 2, and 3):* If you are preparing an NIH grant, many types of expenses are not covered in the categories previously listed, so they are grouped under "other." For example, you might need to purchase the rights to a data collection instrument, pay incentives to subjects, hire transcription services, cover tuition for research assistants, or pay for the analysis of laboratory specimens or long-distance calls or postage for a large survey. Some agencies relegate some of these costs to your institution, so read the FOA and its associated rules carefully and be sure to talk with the budget folks at your institution.

Table 12.2 is a worksheet with examples of expense categories that may help you form your budget.

TABLE 12.2 Example Budget Categories for a 2-Year Budget

Budget categories (Using NIH SF424R&R)	base salary	Year 1 person months	Year 1 salary requested	Year 1 fringe benefits	Year 1 total	base salary	Year 2 person months	Year 2 salary requested	Year 2 fringe benefits	Year 2 total
A. Senior/Key Personnel										
Principal Investigator (academic year)										
Principal Investigator (summer)										
Coinvestigator 1										
Coinvestigator 2										
Statistician										
Total										
B. Other Personnel	base salary	person months	salary requested	fringe benefits	total	base salary	person months	salary requested	fringe benefits	total
Data Collector										
Interventionist										
Data Coder										
Programmer										
Total										
C. Equipment (only use if equipment is > $5,000)										
Total										
D. Travel		# trips	distance	mileage rate	total		# trips	distance	mileage rate	total
Data collection travel										
Intervention travel		registra-tion	travel	per diem	total		registra-tion	travel	per diem	total
Conference travel - conference # 1										
Conference travel - conference # 2										
Total										
E. Participant/Trainee Support Costs (only use if supporting trainees/participants)										
Total										

Budget categories (using NIH SF424R&R)	Year 1			Year 2		
	# of units	cost per unit	total	# of units	cost per unit	total
F. Other Direct Costs						
1. Materials and Supplies						
Computer(s) (must be well justified)						
Printer(s) (must be well justified)						
Computer supplies (toner, flash drive, CDs, paper)						
Stationery & envelopes (for consent letters)						
Digital recorders						
Copying						
Software						
Intervention supplies (booklets, etc.)						
Laboratory supplies						
Cortisol kits						
Blood drawing supplies						
Blood processing supplies						
etc.						
Total						
2. Publication Costs						
(to publish findings/distribute results)						
Total						

	daily rate	# of days	travel	per diem	Total Costs		daily rate	# of days	travel	per diem	Total Costs
3. Consultant Services											
Expert consultant #1											
Total											

4. ADP/Computer Services							
Total							

	Direct Costs	Indirect/F&A Costs	Total Costs		Direct Costs	Indirect/F&A Costs	Total Costs
5. Subawards/Consortium/Contractual Costs							
(only include if someone at another site is a collaborator and contributing to the science)							
Subcontract #1:							
Subcontract #2:							
Total							

(continued)

TABLE 12.2 Example Budget Categories for a 2-Year Budget (*continued*)

Budget categories (using NIH SF424R&R)	Year 1	Year 2
6. **Equipment or Facility Rental/User Fees** (only include if you are paying to use a site or equipment)		
Total		
7. **Alterations and Renovations** (don't include)		
8. **Other 1**		
Books for courses (if you are a fellow/trainee)		
Tuition and fees for you (if you are a fellow/trainee)		
Total		
9. **Other 2**		
Survey/instrument purchase		
Long distance calls		
Postage		
Incentives		
Transcription services		
Specimen analysis fees		
Total		
10. **Other 3**		
Tuition for research assistant (if applicable)		
Total		
a. Total Direct Costs		
b. Base for F&A (Indirect costs)		
c. F&A (Indirect Costs) (% of base)		
d. Total Budget Request (Total Direct Costs plus F&A)		

– *F&A costs:* Once you have tallied the costs of conducting the research (these are called "direct" costs), find out from your institution which of these direct costs serve as the base for calculating the F&A (or indirect, overhead) costs. The base often excludes things such as equipment, subcontract costs in excess of $25,000, and tuition for student research assistants. For research grants, apply the negotiated rate for F&A to the base. For NIH grants where a lower F&A rate is specified, often the total direct costs are used as the base. Be sure to talk to the budget folks at your institution to determine how to calculate the F&A costs.

Once you have gone through this process, it is important to review what has been done and revise as needed; remember also to revise the budget as you revise the methods of your research, so the two are in sync. If you find that you exceed the cap allowed by the FOA, you will need to revise the budget to see whether you can bring it within the guidelines. If you are seeking small funding for preliminary work, remember that often, in the early stages of research, investigators take no salary so that all of the money can be put toward the conduct of the research. But the investigators must commit the time needed for the research or it will not get done successfully. Perhaps, you can compensate coinvestigators for their time by supporting their participation on subsequent larger grants or coauthoring articles with them that report the results of your research. (Negotiate these up front and put them in writing so there are no misunderstandings!)

Budget Justification

The NIH asks you to provide a budget justification to accompany the budget. This is where you explain why you are asking for the specific funds that are in your budget. This section is separate from the budget and details each person's time (specified in person months) and each of the nonpersonnel categories. For each person, say exactly what she or he will do for the project in the time requested; for each nonpersonnel expense, elaborate on why it is needed. Use the same order as in the budget, detail the expenses for the first year, and show your calculations. Then say whether and how subsequent years will differ from the first year.

Modular Budgets

For smaller NIH research budgets (less than $250,000 in all years), the NIH uses what is called a "modular budget." Modular budgets only ask the applicant to specify how much money is needed in increments of $25,000 (a "module"). A modified, shorter budget justification is provided (justifying personnel, subcontracts, and uneven "module" requests across years). However, a caveat is in order: Just because this is all that the NIH needs, it is not necessarily all you should prepare. You need to be certain that you can conduct the research with the money requested, so you may wish first to create a detailed budget and then form it into a modular budget. In addition (a) your institution might want to see a detailed budget before approving the modular budget, and (b) the NIH may wish to see the details before they fund you. Thus, calculating a detailed budget may serve you well, even when all the funder wants at application time is a summary of that budget.

Career Development Award (CDA) Budgets

While the budgets for CDAs are less than $250,000 in all years, they do not employ the type of modular budget outlined earlier. For the NIH, you are asked to put the stipend for yourself (the candidate) under personnel— remembering that you usually need to devote 75% of your time to the project year round, but without going over the maximum allowed by the program to which you are applying. If 75% of your year-round salary doesn't fit within the maximum, you should explain how the additional money you are paid will be covered. Consider stating this in the budget justification and then having your chairperson and dean agree to this in the letter they will sign. Note that fringe benefits on the salary requested in the budget are *not* included in the maximum allowed—they are above and beyond the maximum.

The NIH asks that all of the research and training expenses be totaled and put in Other Direct Costs. Here, too, a maximum is usually specified for the type of award you are seeking, and you need to make sure you do not go over that amount. How do you figure out how much you will need to accomplish your research and training activities? Use the guidelines previously provided to create the budget for your research project, then add expenses related to your training. Will there be tuition costs? Fees? Laboratory costs? Lump all of these into the total you specify, making sure not to go over the maximum allowed. Let us say you are interested in applying for a K01 funded by the National Institute of Nursing Research (NINR). Currently, the NINR funds K01s at $50,000 salary per year for the candidate (plus fringe benefits!) and $20,000 for research and training expenses. For the K23 (the patient-oriented award), the NINR covers $75,000 of your salary per year (plus fringe benefits) and $25,000 in research and training expenses. Other institutes have different maxima, so you may want to check out what each institute offers by clicking on "Table of IC-Specific Information, Requirements and Staff Contacts" in the FOA. And, one caveat: Even though you only need to provide a total for research and training expenses, we would recommend that you create a detailed budget for yourself so you know the project can be done with the total amount requested. Before submitting a proposal, you want to be sure that you can accomplish what you are proposing!

The NIH specifies that the indirect costs (F&A) for CDAs are 8%. Since this is in writing, most institutions adhere to the requirement without fuss. However, some institutions are not happy about the F&A being so low, so be sure to discuss this with your chairperson or dean before doing all the work of writing a proposal that they may not support. CDAs are great ways to get the training you need and to get your research started, so hopefully your institution will support your CDA efforts, especially if you plan to follow up with further proposal funding at the same institution.

Other agencies have varying budgetary requirements for the CDAs though they are similar enough to the NIH guidelines that you can use the NIH guidelines to develop a budget for any CDA. However, be sure to check the guidelines for the program to which you are applying.

Fellowship Budgets

One of the wonderful things about submitting a National Research Service Award (NRSA) pre- or postdoctoral application is that no budget is required for these applications! The amount of the stipend you get and the institutional allowance that the institution gets for your research expenses and training costs are determined each year and specified in an NIH notice that is posted on their webpage (go to the NIH website at www.nih.gov, click on the "Grants and Funding" link, and then on the left-hand side of the page click on "Types of Grant Programs" and then on "Research Training and Fellowships [T and F series]"). This series of clicks will take you right to the NRSA webpage, and by scrolling down you will see links to the stipend levels for each fiscal year. Please note, however, that you *are* asked to provide an estimate of tuition and fees for your training. You will have the opportunity to adjust these just before funding ("Just in Time"), but even then, you won't be paid the full amount of the tuition and fees. Although you specify the total amount of your anticipated tuition and fees, the rule currently is that successful predoctoral applicants receive 60% of the tuition and fees that are requested, up to $16,000 per year, while successful postdoctoral applicants receive 60% of tuition and fees, up to $4,500 per year (different rules are in place for special circumstances, so please read the guidelines). The difference in the maximum tuition and fees paid should tell you that the NIH is expecting less coursework for the postdoctoral applicants than for the predoctoral applicants.

The NIH indicates that there will be *no* indirect costs on fellowship awards, so the institution is supporting you in your pre- or postdoctoral training, with only the institutional allowance that they share with you. Be grateful!

For non-NIH fellowships, be sure to check the guidelines for the agency to which you are applying. Many of these agencies have requirements that are quite similar to those of the NIH, so with luck there won't be many surprises.

Small Research Grant Budgets

If you are applying for a small grant before going to the NIH, the budget is often quite easy to do; see Table 12.3 for an example. Here, the expenses are so limited that the justification for each one is briefly specified right in the budget. You can use the NIH guidelines given previously to think through the types of expenses you might have, but then put the information in whatever format the agency requires. Some agencies have a form you fill out with this information, while others allow you to specify your own format. Their instructions will tell you whether to put the information in the text or perhaps in an appendix, and if you are lucky they will specify in writing the rate for indirect costs and whether those costs are in addition to the allowed budget or included within the budget itself (we say "lucky" because most institutions will accept indirect cost rates that are specified in writing). Always follow their guidelines and never ask for more money than the program allows. In the example we provide in Table 12.3, the proposal is for a $10,000 grant (and thus the direct costs add up to less than $10,000) and the indirect costs, which are limited to 8% but are based on the total direct costs, are added to the total.

You still have to decide whether the project can be done successfully within the parameters of what the agency will fund—do not ask for something that cannot be done. Some folks submit several grants in the hopes that at least one will be awarded or in the hopes of combining several sources of funding to meet the expenses of a project. Unless a funder indicates otherwise, this is allowable as long as you provide full disclosure about your requests and you are not double dipping (having multiple agencies pay for the same expenses). You might submit several proposals for the same expenses and choose only one of the grants if multiple ones are awarded. Or you may want to request funding for different activities from different agencies. This way, you can combine multiple funding sources. However, do not leave reviewers wondering "What will she or he do if not all of the grants are funded?"—articulate plans for these situations (e.g., have you arranged for people to contribute time if needed? Will you be lent equipment? Will laboratory costs be covered by another project if need be?) In addition, managing multiple grants can be challenging. So be careful what you ask for—you just might get it!

Educational Training Project Budgets

The categories of expenses for educational training projects are very similar to those outlined earlier for research projects. The main difference is that you must think through the expenses required to do the educational project, not a research project. In the Personnel section, Who will teach the program(s)? Who will register students for the programs? Will someone be

TABLE 12.3 Sample Simple Budget

Category	Explanation	Dollars
Personnel	Data Entry/Management RA: 80 hours (2 hrs × 40 subjects) @ $15	$1,200.00
	Intervention Nurse: 160 hours (2 home visits × 4 hrs × 20 subjects) @ $25	$4,000.00
		$5,200.00
Supplies	Research supplies (disks, toner, paper, file folders, etc.)	$75.00
	Copying: questionnaires (40 pages/subject), flyers, letters, etc.	$200.00
	NVivo software	$600.00
	Nutrition literature for subjects	$400.00
		$1,275.00
Equipment		$0.00
Travel	Intervention travel to subjects' homes: 2 visits × 60 mi/round trip × 20 subjects @ $0.50	$1,200.00
Computer Costs		$0.00
Other	Subject Incentives: $50 × 40 subjects	$2,000.00
	Postage: 2 mailings × 40 subjects @ $0.60	$48.00
	Long-distance reminder calls for data collection and intervention (80 @ $0.25)	$20.00
		$2,068.00
Total Direct Costs		$9,743.00
Indirect Costs	8% × direct costs	$779.00
Total Costs		$10,522.00

RA, research assistant.

assisting the teachers? Will someone be needed to collect evaluation data? Supplies, equipment, local travel costs, contractual costs, and so forth, all need to be thought through and estimated.

And although some research grants require a match, it is a frequent feature of educational project budgets: People writing proposals for educational projects are often required to split the costs between what they are requesting and what they will get from another source. So be sure to check whether this is required and solicit the funds from the other source(s) prior to writing the full educational proposal—these solicitations can take time!

Often the funds you seek are greater in the early years of an educational project and you plan for them to fade away over the years because the goal of the grant is to help get the program off the ground; it must become more self-sustainable over time. The Health Resources and Services Administration (HRSA), for example, expects you to indicate increasing ability to carry out the program without its help—by reducing the budget each year. Perhaps the program will be integrated into the institution's regular offerings with tuition and fees supporting the program.

APPROVALS

Every institution we can think of and almost all grant programs require institutional approval prior to submission of a proposal. But what is the institution approving? Is it reviewing and approving the science of your proposal? No. The educational program? Possibly. Typically, they are reviewing for several key things: They want to know (a) whether you are making any promises on behalf of the institution, what those promises are, and whether they can follow through on them; (b) whether you have followed the guidelines of the funding agency; (c) whether your budget adds up correctly; and (d) whether the institution can provide the assurances required by the funder (e.g., a smoke-free workplace). The "promises" part is particularly critical for educational programs that might subsequently be integrated into the institution's curricula.

Therefore, most institutions require approvals from your chairperson and/or dean and the equivalent leaders of others on your investigative team before they will sign off on the proposal and submit it to the agency. Why? Because they expect you to work closely with those leaders and/or at least keep them informed as you develop the project. These people are not likely to know whether, for example, an educational program you propose will be appropriate as a subsequent offering in the particular school(s) or college(s) of which you are a part. So throughout the process, it is important to keep your department/division chairperson informed about what you are doing and what you are requesting. Why? If there are commitments you need from that person, you want her or him to be willing to make them. For example, will you be using grant funds to buy yourself out of some other activity? If so, the chair will need to be supportive of this— you don't want to submit a grant that would not be "doable." In the early days of your research, when you might not be able to incorporate investigator funding into the budget of the grant, your chair may be able to support release time for you so you can get your research off the ground. The chair may also wish to evaluate the budget and/or project to make sure it is a good next step for you. And just as you are speaking with your chair, so too should all of the other investigators on your project speak with their chairs. Keep all chairs informed and involved so there are no surprises at signature time.

REVIEW

Reviewers are usually asked to make a decision on the science of your project before tackling the budget, so that budgetary concerns do not interfere with their evaluation of the science. But remember, the budget and the budget justification are a way to show reviewers how knowledgeable and thoughtful you have been in developing the budget. Can the proposed project be done with the budgetary requests you are making? Are the costs so grossly over- or underestimated that the reviewers question your skills as a principal investigator? In other words, is the budget complete and succinctly justified?

CONCLUSION

Develop your budget carefully and in line with the FOA and the research design and methods or educational project you are proposing. Your goal is to design a budget that is appropriate to the project you plan to conduct with a thoughtfulness and thoroughness that are reflected in the accompanying budget justification. Best of luck with your endeavor!

REFERENCE

National Institutes of Health (NIH). (2014, November). Retrieved from http:// grants.nih.gov/grants/funding/424/index.htm

THIRTEEN

SUPPLEMENTAL MATERIALS

Virtually all types of proposals require supplemental materials and these can include everything from how you will protect the rights of your human or animal subjects, if you have them, to how you will go about monitoring the safety of the subjects and the quality of the data you collect, to your plans for sharing what you develop or find with your project to the facilities and resources available for your project, and so forth. In this chapter, we discuss the major types of things you might want to consider for whatever type of proposal you are writing. However, be sure to read the proposal guidelines carefully because each type of proposal considers different things to be critical parts of the text or perhaps supplementary materials. For example, some proposal guidelines indicate that the protection of human subjects should be covered in the Research Design and Methods section, while others expect it in its own section. Some require that you have institutional review board (IRB) approval before submitting the proposal, while others do not expect this to be done until after the proposal has been reviewed positively. For some, a detailed budget and its justification are included in supplemental materials, while other proposals require this information in an appendix or in its own section as part of the text. So read the guidelines carefully, and include the information requested where it is requested.

PROTECTION OF HUMAN SUBJECTS

Many types of proposals ask you to indicate how you will protect the individuals who take part in your study. This is true for almost all research, career development, fellowship, and evidence-based practice (EBP) proposals. But even if you are proposing to conduct an educational project, you may have human subjects in your work. And, even as the principal investigator (PI) or program director (PD), you may not have the ultimate say in whether those participating in your project are viewed as students or subjects, so many institutions will require that you at least submit the project to the local IRB to get their "say so" about whether the project is exempt from further consideration, as most educational projects are.

The National Institutes of Health (NIH) requirements for the protection of human subjects are quite detailed, so they can serve as a good guide for things to consider in any proposal you are writing. Indeed, the NIH discusses the topic extensively in the supplement to its SF424 (R&R) application guidelines (which you will find on the same page that has the link to the application guidelines [www.grants.nih.gov/grants/funding/424/index.htm]; scroll down—it is the last entry in the box labeled "Instructions for Application Forms"). Lots of information is included about whether you are studying human subjects, whether you are exempt from providing information on the protection of human subjects, whether you are conducting a clinical trial involving human subjects, and so forth. Please read the guidelines carefully.

The NIH requests that you include certain information in the Protection of Human Subjects section. Note that this section overlaps with the Methods section, but is not included in the page limit. Therefore, some people put methods details only here in the Protection of Human Subjects section. We would not recommend doing that. Why? Because by the time the reader gets to this section, she or he has already wondered how the methods issues are going to be addressed and whether you have forgotten them. The reader wants the information where it is first relevant. Therefore, at least mention each of the method details in the Approach section, but if you are lacking space, you can refer the reader to additional details in the Human Subjects section.

The information that the NIH requests in the Protection of Human Subjects section begins with a section called Risks to the Subjects. This section should include information on subjects' involvement and characteristics, the design of the study, the sources of materials about subjects, and the potential risks to subjects. You can see that a lot of methods details are requested, but we would recommend including the details even if they seem to overlap with the Approach section. And, of course, the information should *not* contradict what is in the Approach section; if you have decided to change an aspect of the design, be sure to change it in both places so everything is internally consistent.

The hardest section for some people to write is the Risks section, (a) because it is very hard to present risks without also addressing how you are going to deal with them (the next section focuses on those protections), and (b) also because investigators sometimes have trouble thinking that there is any risk to participating in the study. But what if, for example, agreeing to participate in, let us say, an HIV study means that the person has an HIV diagnosis and that information gets out. There clearly is a risk related to confidentiality (that you are going to work hard to prevent). What if your questions and/or questionnaires have a subject questioning a health decision she or he has made or increases her or his fear? What if you are discussing end-of-life issues for folks who are seriously ill but who have spent all their energy staying alive and now wonder if they are dying? What if you ask parents of premature infants with cardiovascular problems whether they or others in the family have or have had cardiovascular problems? Is there a chance you will increase potential guilt? What about elders who might be at risk because of extreme exhaustion while participating in your study? And so on. Think through your methods and do the very best you can to minimize any possible risks. You get to talk about ways you are minimizing risks in the next section, but you need to elaborate on the potential risks here.

The second section is Adequacy of Protection Against Risks, and this section should include your plans for recruitment and informed consent and protection against risks. The NIH wants to be sure that you will be recruiting subjects in an informed and nonbiased manner (no coercion, please!), that you will seek truly informed consent, that you will document that consent, and that your study will be conducted in a way that protects subjects from risks or minimizes those risks. Be sure to discuss any special plans you are putting in place to deal with particularly vulnerable populations (e.g., pregnant women, prisoners, infants, or other children) and document how you will help subjects who experience adverse events during any intervention you are studying.

The third section is Potential Benefits of the Proposed Research to the Subjects and Others. There may be no benefits to the subjects in your study, and it is okay to say this if it is true. But think it through before saying that there are no benefits. Perhaps participation in your study will offer subjects a chance to express opinions that they might otherwise not get to share with others. Perhaps you will be providing psychological support to subjects during a difficult health crisis. Or perhaps you will be providing health care or regular monitoring that subjects would not get if they did not participate in your study. (Note that monetary incentives or compensation that you will provide to subjects generally should not be included as a benefit.) Lastly, indicate why you think the risks are reasonable in relation to the anticipated benefits.

The fourth section is Importance of the Knowledge to Be Gained. You are proposing to do the study for a reason, and that reason needs to be shown to be compelling in the rationale for the study. So look back to what you wrote there and paraphrase it for this section. Here, however, you will also include information about why the risks to subjects are reasonable in relation to the knowledge to be gained. Note that this is not the same thing as the risk/benefit ratio for an individual subject, but the risk for subjects in relation to the knowledge to be gained from the study as a whole.

The NIH understands that you will work through your local IRB, so be sure to say that you will, but the NIH usually does not require that you include your consent forms or, for that matter, IRB approval of the project until it is about to be funded. This is not true for all types of proposals you might be preparing or submitting, especially for proposals related to seeking a degree, so please read carefully and follow the guidelines for proposals from the agency to which you will be submitting.

A word about "delayed onset" human subjects: Sometimes you will submit a proposal long before you are ready to start the study. Heck, the research design and methods might even change before you start the study because you are going to receive important training before the study is undertaken. This is particularly true for proposals like those for predoctoral or postdoctoral fellowships and career development awards. When you are in a situation where funding will start before your study is to be done, you may want to request "delayed onset" human subjects designation. This means that you do not have to specify all of the details right this minute, but you will need to do so *prior* to beginning the study. All of the rules related to protecting human subjects still apply, they are just delayed a bit until you are ready to start the study. You still *must* submit the human subjects section to the NIH and get local IRB approval prior to conducting the study, but you do not need to do these things at the time the proposal is submitted (or funded).

Data and Safety Monitoring

No matter what sort of project you are proposing, if you are collecting data (and you should be), you need to have detailed plans in the Methods section to ensure the quality of the data obtained throughout the project. You have heard the old adage: garbage in, garbage out. If you have sloppy data collection methods, you will have garbage. So have detailed plans for how the data will be collected: how you will train data collectors to standardize their procedures, how you will regularly monitor the collection of data, and what you will do if that monitoring detects problems. If you see problems, plan to fix them right away so that you are comfortable with your data and the validity of your results.

Just as you monitor the quality of the data you are collecting, you also need to monitor the safety of the subjects you have in your project. This might not be needed for some educational projects, but it is needed for all research projects that are evaluating interventions. If you are not proposing an intervention study, technically you do not need to monitor subject safety, but we would recommend that you at least consider whether your study methods might affect subjects and, if so, describe your plans to monitor subjects, identify problems, and solve them.

If you are evaluating an intervention, what do you need to have? Read the guidelines and follow what is requested. In general, the monitoring required will need to match the level of risk to subjects and the size and complexity of the study. The greater the size and complexity or the greater the risk, the more rigorous the monitoring needs to be. At the simplest level, you need to present a data and safety monitoring (DSM) plan, including the persons who will do the monitoring, the procedures for doing so, and the process for timely adverse event identification and reporting. As risk, size, and complexity increase, so does the need for independent, in-depth monitoring. Often, when you are fully testing the efficacy of an intervention (perhaps via an R01 at the NIH), you will be required to have a data and safety monitoring board (DSMB) perform this function. While the thought of creating such a board can be rather daunting, fear not, for your institution's IRB might have such a board available to help you. Stay calm, plan carefully, document that planning in what you write, see how your institution might help you, and then *follow through*.

Inclusion of Women and Minorities

Your goal in designing a study is to be as inclusive and representative as possible. Do not try to generalize from men to women, from Whites to non-Whites, from adults to children, and so forth. Populations differ from one another, and each might respond in unique ways to your intervention or study methods. While you do not have to study everyone in one study (you want to control as much as you can!), you should have a strong rationale for why you are choosing to study those that you are. This section should be included for any studies involving human subjects and should address four things: subject selection criteria and your rationale for the inclusion of genders and ethnicities/races, your rationale for the exclusion of any gender or ethnic/racial group, your proposed outreach programs for recruiting gender and ethnic/racial groups, and a planned enrollment report.

Planned Enrollment Report

The planned enrollment report is not used for collecting data from potential subjects, but it is a very good way to lay out the gender, ethnicity, and racial makeup of your anticipated subjects. We have included a copy of the NIH's Planned Enrollment Report here (Table 13.1), but you can always access

TABLE 13.1 NIH Planned Enrollment Report

Racial Categories	Ethnic Categories				
	Not Hispanic or Latino		Hispanic or Latino		
	Female	Male	Female	Male	Total
American Indian/Alaska Native					0
Asian					0
Native Hawaiian or other Pacific Islander					0
Black or African American					0
White					0
More than one race					0
Total	0	0	0	0	0

From the NIH (2012).

the latest version in the additional format pages section that accompanies the SF424 (R&R) application (www.grants.nih.gov/grants/funding/424/index.htm#format). Complete the table and include it in your application. The table should match what you say in the text of your application, so make sure they parallel one another!

A few comments are in order. The only ethnicity the NIH focuses on at this time is Hispanic/Latino. The NIH wants to know how many female and male Hispanic/Latinos and non-Hispanic/Latinos individuals you plan to study. You are also required to designate a racial category for each person; and, no, Hispanic/Latino is not a race, it is an ethnicity, so each person of each gender will have both an ethnicity and a race. This can be problematic when your sites give you data about potential subjects that specify Hispanic as a race, but you must work through those data to try to determine a race for each possible subject. You do not want to make up your projected numbers or over guestimate the numbers you will have—you will be held accountable for recruiting the numbers you indicate, so be honest and have a strong rationale for your exclusion criteria.

Are you expected to have both genders and all races? Not necessarily. You do not want to exclude an important group just because they are not in your locale (you could collaborate with someone else who has access to the group), but populations that are in your locale might be most important to study. Make a case for whatever groups you decide to include or exclude and design the study so that you have sufficient numbers of individuals to test your hypotheses or answer your research questions for each important subgroup.

Inclusion of Children

The NIH is also interested in making sure that children are included in studies, as appropriate. If your goal is to generalize to children, you should be studying them; but if you are studying something that is not appropriate for children (perhaps a gerontological topic?), it is okay not to include them if you explain your rationale. Note that the NIH considers anyone under the age of 21 as a child, so you might be studying children if you are including subjects age 18 and older. You should always include this section if you are studying human subjects. If children are included, be sure to read about and address the additional protections that are required (e.g., will you be getting parental/guardian consent and child assent to participate in the study?).

VERTEBRATE ANIMALS

What if you are not using human subjects or their tissues but animal subjects in your proposed study? If that is the case, there are all sorts of assurances you must provide if you are using vertebrate animals (e.g., mice, rats, rabbits). You are expected to describe the animals and justify their use, provide information on their veterinary care, indicate procedures for their protection, and discuss any plans for euthanasia. Just as your institution probably has an IRB for human subjects, it probably also has an Institutional Animal Care and Use Committee (IACUC) that may be able to guide you in the preparation of this material and, of course, it will need to approve your study prior to its conduct.

SELECT AGENT RESEARCH

While few nursing studies use select agents (toxins and other hazardous biological agents), it is certainly not unheard of for nursing and other health care studies to include them. If you are using them in your studies, be sure to follow all state and federal laws for their safe use and, in this section, identify the agents you will use and provide registration information and descriptions of the sites where you will be using them. Read the details of what is required in this section and follow them carefully.

MULTIPLE PD/PI LEADERSHIP PLAN

Nowadays, when projects are quite complex or large, there is often more than one "leader" of the project. While in prior days, people referred to PI and co-PI or PD, the NIH recognizes that multiple people might be leading a project and currently uses the term "multiple" PIs or PDs. But when there are multiple people leading a project, there are all sorts of leadership issues that might occur, so you are asked to draft a leadership plan as a part of preparing the proposal. It is this plan that you put in this section. Present your rationale for choosing multiple people to lead the project and indicate how things will be structured so you can work well together. How will you communicate? How will decisions be made about scientific issues? How will differences be resolved? And how will resources be distributed? Cover all of these things and any others that are relevant to your particular situation.

CONSORTIUM/CONTRACTUAL ARRANGEMENTS

When scientists at institutions other than your own are participating on your scientific team, your institution usually needs to form consortia or have some sort of contractual agreements with their institution(s). (This is not the case when people are serving as your consultants and are not representing their institutions.) While the details of budgets and their justifications are covered in the Budget section, your goal in this section is to provide a brief overview of what team members' involvement will be; often a letter formalizing the arrangements is included. (Note that consortial arrangements are not needed when the institution involved in your study does not have someone participating on your scientific team. For example, you might have sites that allow you to access their patients but no one from those institutions is on your investigative team.) Be careful that the tail is not wagging the dog—if it looks like the consortial institution is doing more than you are, the question may be raised as to why you and your institution are serving in the primary role—why isn't the consorital institution? Use this space to explain why you and your institution are primary if the consortial institution will play a significant role in the project.

LETTERS OF SUPPORT

There are a number of different kinds of letters of support you might need for your project. You will put some of these in an appendix (see the "Appendices" section of this chapter), but some are mandated to be included either as part of the proposal or in a Letters of Support section. For the NIH, typically letters of support from settings or sites where you will identify subjects, intervene, or collect data are included in an appendix. But if you have individuals on your team who are serving as consultants, consortium participants, or collaborators, you put their letters together in a Letters of Support section. (Note that you do *not* need letters from individuals who will be staff on a project [e.g., research assistants].) It is particularly important that these letters spell out what the arrangements are for participation on your project. For many, if not most, this might include details about co-authorship of articles or presentations emanating from the research (yes, you should discuss these things early on). Consultant letters should also include the number of hours/days/weeks they anticipate being involved each year of the project, fees to be charged, and how the consultation will be provided. (Will the person travel to your site? Will the consultation be via Skype? Will it be done via e-mail? Will you meet at conferences? Will it be a mixture of these things?) Collaborators who are in charge of a facility you will be using in your study should say what resources will be provided and what sort of access you will have. If there is a fee for such services, it should be noted and the information should parallel what you present in your budget and budget justification.

You want all of these letters to make positive statements about the proposed research and what they can contribute to it. How do you go about getting this? You might want to draft the letters for these people so each can give an accurate paragraph about the study and its importance. Just be sure that you write a slightly different letter for each person or it will be clear to the reviewers that you wrote the letters! You also might want to ask these people to sing their own praises in terms of what they (or their facility) will bring to the project. But be sure that this information parallels what is presented in the biosketch and does not undermine you as the PI. Therefore, read each letter carefully, and yes, you can ask the individual to rewrite sections if needed.

Many institutions have their own rules about what roles people can play on your project. For example, someone you are interested in including on your team who is within your institution may not be able to be called a consultant—that term might be reserved for people outside of your institution. So you might need to get creative in terms of what you "call" various people (co-PI, co-investigator, investigator, statistical investigator, collaborating investigator, etc.).

Should you have letters of support from your chairperson and/or dean? Many do this, but we don't see the need for such letters unless they are requested (e.g., for Career Development Awards). Why? These folks are going to be quite positive about you and your research, and typically you will write the letters for them, so what purpose do they serve?

Non-NIH research proposals may have specific guidelines they would like you to follow in terms of letters of support, and be sure to allow enough time to obtain all the requested letters.

RESOURCE SHARING PLANS (OR PLANS FOR DISSEMINATION OF MODEL AND FINDINGS)

Most funders want to be sure that the projects they are supporting will reach their intended audiences and not just via the typical presentations and publications (although these are also important!). For example, if you did a study in the community, you want to present the outcomes to the community and discuss ways that useful aspects of the project can be continued. If you developed a model for providing case management in schools for children with chronic illnesses, you want to make the approach available to school nurses. If you have developed a model for helping nursing home staff end the use of antipsychotic drugs for residents with dementia, make it widely available. And if you have developed a new educational training program, describe how you will make the approach and the materials available to others.

Products of your work might include everything from the results of your project to innovations you develop along the way (e.g., model organisms, genomic analyses, methods, measures, interventions). Some things always must be shared (model organisms and large genomic analyses), so be sure to read the guidelines carefully and follow them. In other cases, the need for sharing may depend on the amount of funding or the requirements of the funding opportunity announcement (FOA). For example, a Data Sharing Plan in which you specify what data you will share and how you will share it is required at certain levels of funding and by certain FOAs. Will you send data CDs to people, or perhaps put the data on a secure website? Will you require that people "apply" to you or someone at your institution to use the data? Will you require that they follow rules for the ethical conduct of research? And so forth.

Before sharing data, be sure to clean the data and take out identifiers of all types. Of course it is assumed that you will include a codebook and an overview of the study along with the data. Some institutions have begun helping investigators by having local resources to assist in the planning and implementation of data sharing. Whatever you do, please make sure that you share the data in a timely manner, because "old" data are not really worth much. If you will be able to share the data during a grant's funding period and you have expenses related to that sharing, you can usually include them in your budget. However, if you are conducting a small study or one in which subjects might be identifiable from their combined individual factors, you may wish to say that you cannot share the data and explain why.

FACILITIES AND OTHER RESOURCES (INCLUDING EQUIPMENT)

Every project requires some sort of facilities, resources, and/or equipment to support its conduct. Most proposal guidelines specify that you should describe what your proposed project will have available in the way of these supports. Do not, however, include a generic list of every facility available on your campus. That is *not* what most proposals are asking you to include. Instead, most proposal guidelines ask you to describe the facilities, resources, and equipment that are relevant and available to support your project. Think about institutes and centers in your institution or nearby that are particularly relevant to your work and with which you have made arrangements to support your work. What about computer resources? Library resources? Clinical resources? Do you need access to a particular laboratory and its equipment? Will such a laboratory be available to you? Perhaps your research project will require access to a laboratory that can provide a special freezer in which to store your biological samples. Perhaps you say you have access to accelerometers.

If you propose an educational training project, it is important to talk about your school's and university's capacities and the support they will provide the project. Health Resources and Services Administration (HRSA) guidelines tell you what kind of information they want, so provide it. For example, will students need and have access to a simulation lab? Technological support for distance education?

Reviewers will be looking at your description of the facilities and other resources and equipment to determine whether these are available to you, and at your letters of support to make sure that the plans are solidified. Therefore, be sure to "personalize" the facilities and resources you describe—say how you will use them in the study and have the letters parallel this information. If you will not be using a resource, don't include it!

BIBLIOGRAPHY AND REFERENCES CITED

Virtually every application will require you to include a list of the sources you cite in the text—the foundation for your proposed work. This may be called Reference List, Literature Cited, Bibliography, or some other name (e.g., the NIH calls this section Bibliography and References Cited). Unlike some lists, this typically is *not* a list of everything you have read. Instead, it is a list of the relevant literature you have cited for making the case for your study, the theory or conceptualization you have chosen to guide your work, the instruments you will be using and their psychometrics, methodological or statistical approaches that are not well known, and so forth. If you cite a source anywhere in the text, including in a table or figure, be sure to include the reference for the citation in this list. This list may have some limits imposed by the funder in the application guidelines (such as "be no longer than four pages")—so be sure to check.

Some funders have a specific format they would like you to follow in preparing this list. It might be in the style of the American Psychological Association (APA), the American Medical Association, the National Library of Medicine, and so forth, but most ask that you choose a style and stick with it—be complete and consistent in what you present. When you retrieve articles from online resources, they may come to you in many different formats, so you are asked to make everything internally consistent; do not have the dates or page numbers in different places for different references. Also, if you use some sort of reference software while you are preparing an application (a) you may want to use an expansive citation style in the text to start with (such as APA) so you get the references correct and then change to a more condensed format (such as a numbering style) at the end—especially if you are short on space; (b) usually you should unlink the citations from the references before you submit the application; and (c) make sure to check the final copy so you are certain that the text citations match up with the correct references in the list. This last point is key, because you do not want to submit the wrong references to the funder!

APPENDICES

It is very important for you to follow the guidelines provided for the project you are submitting. If you are told not to include appendices, do not include them. If you are told not to use the appendices as a way to get around text limitations, do not do it. If you are told not to put tables or figures that belong in the text in the appendices, do not do it! Do not just assume that you can squeeze things in; reviewers won't like you, if you get that far—you might just be tossed out in the preview stage if you do not follow the rules. Learn the rules and follow them.

For Research, Career Development Award, and Fellowship Proposals

For most research, career development award, and fellowship proposals, appendices are allowed. Why? Because they can be very informative to the reviewers. For example, you may not have enough space to describe each instrument in detail, but you may be able to put the actual instruments in the appendix thereby providing reviewers with information they might not otherwise have had.

It is usually helpful to group your appendix materials into a few key appendices, to put a summary sheet at the front of the entire set of appendices with your name and listing each appendix and what its focus is, and then to begin each appendix with a cover sheet that lists what is in that appendix. The order of what you present should match the text so the reader does not have the rifle through the information to find what she or he needs. A common organization of this material is:

- Appendix A: Support Letters
- Appendix B: Intervention Protocols
- Appendix C: Instruments
- Appendix D: Publications

If you are submitting a grant to the NIH, the support letters mentioned for Appendix A are meant to be support letters from individuals or organizations other than your investigative team (consultant letters go in another place). For example, in the Setting section, you might have said that you will recruit subjects from Settings A, B, and C, and conduct the project in Setting D. Letters from A, B, C, *and* D should be put in this section. All of these letters should be on appropriate letterhead, signed by an appropriate individual, and enthusiastic about your project. Letters from A, B, and C should talk about their facilities and how many clients they serve like the individuals you wish to study; the letter from D should describe the access you will be provided to the facilities you need to conduct your study. To help these people out, you can (and should) write the letters for them, but please make sure that they are not identical so reviewers do not know that you have written them.

Intervention protocols are important to include if you have an intervention: They can provide details to buttress what is in the text. Do you have to have developed protocols for all of your intervention sessions? You should have them if you have done preliminary studies on the intervention—if not, reviewers will wonder why not. If you are in the early stages of developing an intervention, you might want to give an example protocol in detail and then provide overviews of others. What goes into such a protocol? Everything from the content to be covered, to its organization, notes on delivery, and so forth. You are basically showing how you will operationalize the details you put in the text of the application.

Appendix C includes all of the instruments that you will use in your study in the same order they are discussed in the text. Just clump them together, but for heaven's sake, do not take off the instrument names or run all of the items together as you might ultimately do for subjects. Why? Because readers will have no clue which instrument is which. Leave the instruments in their original forms and leave the names on them so readers can flip through the appendices while reading the corresponding text. What if something is not an "instrument" but perhaps instead is a physiological measure? Put the protocol for how you will go about assessing the physiological measure in place of the instrument. If you are collecting a biological sample? Ditto (and, by the way, be sure to include a letter in Appendix A from the laboratory that will do your analysis). What if you plan to conduct a semistructured interview? Put a list of the interview questions here. Thus, this appendix should be a comprehensive collection of instruments and protocols you will use to collect your data.

Appendix D is usually reserved for publications of the PI, but each agency has its own rules about what you can include, so be sure to study them carefully. For example, the NIH has changed its rules so that only up to three publications may be included, and publications may only be included if they are not publicly available. Within those two rules, the NIH will typically accept manuscripts or abstracts that are accepted for publication or that are published but not available via a free, publicly available online link. Why these limits? There simply is not a need to include copies of articles that readers can get access to in other ways. Also, when 10 publications were allowed, everyone put a full 10 articles including ones that were from co-investigators or even ones that were not relevant to the application being submitted.

If there is other information you wish to include in the appendices (e.g., informed consent documents), feel free to do so as long as you follow the rules set forth by the agency to which you are submitting. Use appendices to buttress the text, not to circumvent it!

For HRSA Grant Proposals

If you are submitting a HRSA grant proposal, you need to provide at least 11 attachments (and possibly 12) in your appendix. We briefly summarize these as follows. Remember that you have only 80 pages total for the application, and these attachments are part of those 80 pages, so be as brief as you can. Once you have put the attachments together, you may need to go back and condense, or cut, to be sure you are not over the limit—or taking up the space needed to present essential elements of the program in your narrative.

Attachment #1 is a description of the program you are proposing, the focus of the program, and projected student enrollment figures for each year of the program. Attachment #2 should include all letters of agreement and memorandums of agreement between your school or college and the organizations you will work with. Attachment #3 is an official letter of accreditation of your school or college, signed and dated by the accrediting body. However, for new programs, your school can be considered accredited if there is reason to believe that you will meet accreditation standards by the beginning of the academic year following graduation of the first students in the program, or if you meet other specified conditions. HRSA provides clear information on the process you must follow with a new program. Attachment #4 provides documentation of approval of new master's or doctoral programs, with meeting minutes, or a letter from the Faculty Senate or from the Board of Regents or Board of Governors, and so forth.

Attachment #5 includes information on the curriculum that trainees will be enrolled in, including course descriptions—which, incidentally, should show how the curriculum meets the requirements for statutory funding preference if you are requesting that. Also, this attachment includes the evidence-based tools to be used to measure trainee competencies. Attachment #6 includes administrative and other letters of support indicating what will be provided to the applicant if the project is funded.

These letters should be from the dean of the school, university officials, and key officials in collaborating organizations.

Attachment #7 provides position descriptions for project personnel, including clinical preceptors. Attachment #8 provides the qualifications and the nature of the work to be done by consultants to the project. And Attachment #9 gives the biosketches of key project personnel (including any key consultants). These biosketches can follow the format used for NIH proposals, but they cannot be more than two pages long.

Attachment #10 gives the baseline expenditures for the school's last fiscal year and an estimate for the next fiscal year, using a chart supplied by HRSA. Finally, if you are seeking the statutory funding preference, Attachment #11 provides the data documenting that you qualify for this: Either graduates serve the underserved or work in rural areas or in health departments. Attachment #12 is for any other information you need to present.

For Other Proposals

Other proposals, such as PhD proposals and EBP project proposals, also include appendices, but their content will depend on the PhD or Doctor of Nursing Practice (DNP) committee or the requirements of the agency approving or funding the proposal. If you are doing a PhD proposal, you may need to include a table providing data on all the studies you have reviewed. Also, whether you are doing a PhD proposal or another type of proposal, your appendices will need to include letters from agencies indicating permission to conduct the study in that setting, a protocol for the intervention if the project includes an intervention, and copies of any instruments to be used in the study. You may also include a manual for training people to carry out the intervention and if you are seeking funding, other materials you deem relevant. Consult your PhD or DNP committee, agency committee, or the funding agency guidelines to see what else may need to be included. And use the NIH guidelines described earlier to help you.

REFERENCE

National Institutes of Health (NIH). (2012, August). *Planned enrollment report*. Retrieved from http://grants.nih.gov/grants/funding/phs398/PlannedEnrollmentReport.pdf

SECTION IV: DEVELOPING, SUBMITTING, AND REVIEWING PROPOSALS: NEXT STEPS

FOURTEEN

DEVELOPING THE PROPOSAL: START TO FINISH

PLANNING A TIMELINE FOR SUBMISSION

To produce a compelling proposal, you will probably need to write at least four drafts and maybe many more. We have suggested a timeline for preparing proposals for funding (Figure 14.1). For a PhD proposal or Doctor of Nursing Practice (DNP) proposal, your timeline may depend in part on your work schedule and other factors in your life, and on the timeline of your chair. But remember, if you are in graduate school, the aim is to propose the work, do it, and graduate, not to spend the rest of your life in school.

In planning any proposal, the key is to work backward from the deadline, noting all things you need to do and deciding when you will do them. Put these decisions on a calendar that shows what you will do when (you can find lots of these calendars on the Internet), and share this calendar with your research team and advisors, as appropriate. When you are developing your calendar, remember holidays. If you need external reviewers for a proposal you plan to submit in February, it is pointless to send it to them on December 15. You have to factor in the long holiday break when many universities are closed and your reviewers are not thinking about your proposal. You might get the reviews back by mid to late January—too late for you to make any substantial revisions.

The NIH standard deadlines are February, June, and October; if you plan to submit in February, you need to be working on the first draft and the logistics of your plan by August; if the deadline is June, by November, and so on. Other funding agencies also have deadlines, and you need the

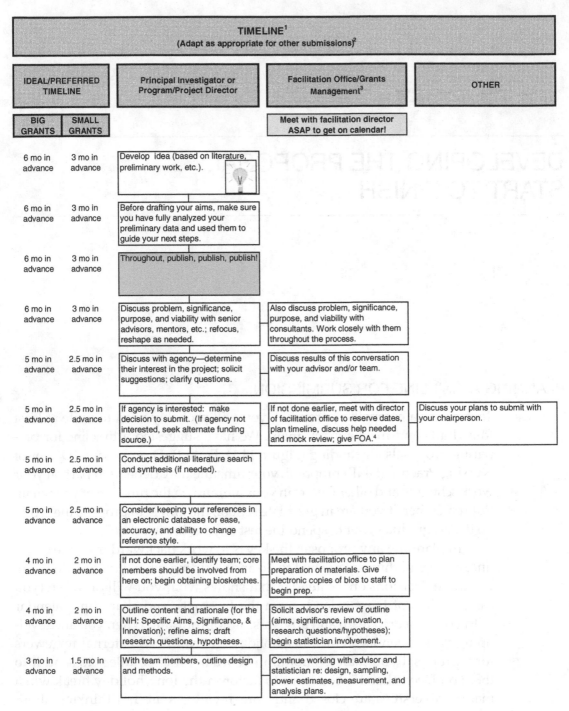

TIMELINE[1] (Adapt as appropriate for other submissions)[2]			
IDEAL/PREFERRED TIMELINE	**Principal Investigator or Program/Project Director**	**Facilitation Office/Grants Management[3]**	**OTHER**

BIG GRANTS	**SMALL GRANTS**		Meet with facilitation director ASAP to get on calendar!	
6 mo in advance	3 mo in advance	Develop idea (based on literature, preliminary work, etc.).		
6 mo in advance	3 mo in advance	Before drafting your aims, make sure you have fully analyzed your preliminary data and used them to guide your next steps.		
6 mo in advance	3 mo in advance	Throughout, publish, publish, publish!		
6 mo in advance	3 mo in advance	Discuss problem, significance, purpose, and viability with senior advisors, mentors, etc.; refocus, reshape as needed.	Also discuss problem, significance, purpose, and viability with consultants. Work closely with them throughout the process.	
5 mo in advance	2.5 mo in advance	Discuss with agency—determine their interest in the project; solicit suggestions; clarify questions.	Discuss results of this conversation with your advisor and/or team.	
5 mo in advance	2.5 mo in advance	If agency is interested: make decision to submit. (If agency not interested, seek alternate funding source.)	If not done earlier, meet with director of facilitation office to reserve dates, plan timeline, discuss help needed and mock review; give FOA.[4]	Discuss your plans to submit with your chairperson.
5 mo in advance	2.5 mo in advance	Conduct additional literature search and synthesis (if needed).		
5 mo in advance	2.5 mo in advance	Consider keeping your references in an electronic database for ease, accuracy, and ability to change reference style.		
4 mo in advance	2 mo in advance	If not done earlier, identify team; core members should be involved from here on; begin obtaining biosketches.	Meet with facilitation office to plan preparation of materials. Give electronic copies of bios to staff to begin prep.	
4 mo in advance	2 mo in advance	Outline content and rationale (for the NIH: Specific Aims, Significance, & Innovation); refine aims; draft research questions, hypotheses.	Solicit advisor's review of outline (aims, significance, innovation, research questions/hypotheses); begin statistician involvement.	
3 mo in advance	1.5 mo in advance	With team members, outline design and methods.	Continue working with advisor and statistician re: design, sampling, power estimates, measurement, and analysis plans.	

FIGURE 14.1 Suggested Timeline for Grant Submission Activities

TIMELINE			
IDEAL/PREFERRED TIMELINE	**Principal Investigator or Program/Project Director**	**Facilitation Office/Grants Management**[3]	**OTHER**
BIG GRANTS / **SMALL GRANTS**			
3 mo in advance / 1.5 mo in advance	Negotiate with sites for access to subjects; get letters of agreement and data on site clients; begin sub-contracts for scientific collaborators.	Give copies of the letters to research office for inclusion in an appendix.	
3 mo in advance / 1.5 mo in advance	Continue writing the proposal; share work among team members; read and edit each other; rewrite as needed.		
3 mo in advance / 1.5 mo in advance	Plan for institutional review board (IRB) review if required by the agency for submission. (The NIH usually does not require prior to submission.)	Your office of human research ethics/IRB can answer questions.	If you will have subcontracting institutions, be sure to get their IRB approvals as well, if required; be sure to stay on top of this.
3 mo in advance / 1.5 mo in advance	From here forward: revise/rewrite based on editorial input and critiques; repeat editing/rewriting steps in 2-week cycles.	Have advisor read as scheduled (give approximately 1 week for each read) and PREARRANGE!	Also have team members continue reading and revising; ask other faculty colleagues to read selectively.
2 mo in advance / 1 mo in advance	Once you have a good sense of the team members, study methods, and timline begin to draft the budget and budget justification.	Meet with grants manager to design budget; grants manager may prepare budget; 3–4 drafts usually needed.	All investigators on grant meet with chairpersons to discuss anticipated percent time commitment to the grant.
2 mo in advance / 1 mo in advance	Begin collecting copies of selected measurement tools for appendix; give these and other materials to facilitation office when ready.		
7 wk in advance	When close to final draft of proposal is ready, give to facilitation office for distribution to mock reviewers.	Facilitation office may arrange the review, distribute copies, and host the review	Give copies to external reviewers if they are to review and provide feedback (payment is usually involved).
6 wk in advance / 3 wk in advance (if needed)	Biosketches, facilities and other resources, key personnel, etc., should be complete by now.		
6 wk in advance / 3 wk in advance, if doing	Have mock review of proposal, including team members, advisor and other reviewers.		
6 wk through 2 wks in advance / 3 wk in advance	Revise/rewrite based on feedback during mock review; count on one or two additional rounds of review by advisor and an editor.	Advisor continues to read as needed; if editor is to read, she or he usually reads the first or second post-mock review draft.	
1 mo in advance / 3 wk in advance	Finalize budget and budget justification; give to facilitation office to review.		

FIGURE 14.1 Suggested Timeline for Grant Submission Activities (*continued*)

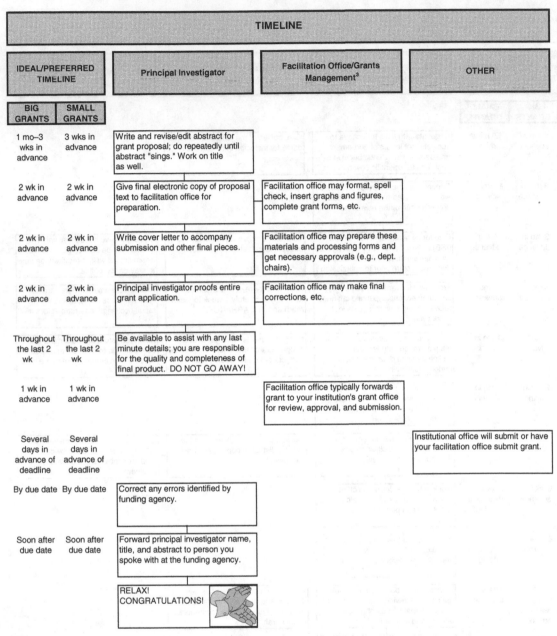

TIMELINE			
IDEAL/PREFERRED TIMELINE	**Principal Investigator**	**Facilitation Office/Grants Management[3]**	**OTHER**
BIG GRANTS / **SMALL GRANTS**			
1 mo–3 wks in advance / 3 wks in advance	Write and revise/edit abstract for grant proposal; do repeatedly until abstract "sings." Work on title as well.		
2 wk in advance / 2 wk in advance	Give final electronic copy of proposal text to facilitation office for preparation.	Facilitation office may format, spell check, insert graphs and figures, complete grant forms, etc.	
2 wk in advance / 2 wk in advance	Write cover letter to accompany submission and other final pieces.	Facilitation office may prepare these materials and processing forms and get necessary approvals (e.g., dept. chairs).	
2 wk in advance / 2 wk in advance	Principal investigator proofs entire grant application.	Facilitation office may make final corrections, etc.	
Throughout the last 2 wk / Throughout the last 2 wk	Be available to assist with any last minute details; you are responsible for the quality and completeness of final product. DO NOT GO AWAY!		
1 wk in advance / 1 wk in advance		Facilitation office typically forwards grant to your institution's grant office for review, approval, and submission.	
Several days in advance of deadline / Several days in advance of deadline			Institutional office will submit or have your facilitation office submit grant.
By due date / By due date	Correct any errors identified by funding agency.		
Soon after due date / Soon after due date	Forward principal investigator name, title, and abstract to person you spoke with at the funding agency.		
	RELAX! CONGRATULATIONS!		

Notes

[1]The timeline for grant preparation cannot be entirely pre-determined. The principal investigator should meet with the appropriate director (in charge of the research office, educational proposals, etc.) early in the process to plan an individualized timeline that takes into account the nature of the proposal, the preparing office's contraints (such as multiple grants being planned for submission at the same time), and the principal investigator's schedule. Research assistants have particularly short turn-around times, so designing an appropriate timeline becomes especially important.

[2]Note that for some proposals (e.g., a career development award or a fellowship), you should work closely with your mentor(s)/sponsor(s).

[3]Some schools assign senior as advisors to individuals submitting grants; use that person throughout your proposal preparation.

[4]FOA, funding opportunity announcement.

FIGURE 14.1 Suggested Timeline for Grant Submission Activities (*continued*)

same advance time for those, so check the guidelines for submission dates as soon as you think about submitting a proposal. People who wait until the last minute to write a proposal are not usually funded; and if you do that, you will have wasted your time and the time of the reviewers.

PUBLISHING PRELIMINARY WORK

If you are writing an NIH proposal (other than a small R03 proposal), you will need a section reporting preliminary work that shows that the study is feasible, you can carry it out as planned, and it is likely to be successful. Other funding agencies also want to know whether you have done work in preparation for what you are proposing. In both cases you must write articles reporting this preliminary work. If you submit a proposal without having published your prior work, your chances of getting funded plummet. For good reason. Why should anyone fund people to do work that they never disseminate and no one ever hears about? We cannot emphasize this enough. While proposal reviewers may read the abstract of a proposal first, many then go straight to your biosketch to see what you have published before they look at anything else, and if they don't see much, they are likely to comment that investigators have not published prior work and give you a bad score. This will be the case for all proposals other than PhD, DNP, and fellowship proposals. (And if you are applying for a fellowship, a publication on your record looks very good; it shows reviewers that you will disseminate your work.)

Therefore, as you look at your timeline for preparing a proposal, give top priority to submitting articles on any prior work you have completed. Did you publish the findings from your dissertation? If it is not too late, do so now. Did you publish the outcomes of your last study? Write those articles now. For the NIH, unless you are writing a National Research Service Award (NRSA) fellowship proposal, you cannot include articles on your biosketch until they are in press (accepted for publication), so you need to write and submit articles early enough to get them accepted. You can note that an article reporting the work is "under review" in your section on preliminary work, but not all reviewers will read that section carefully, though they all carefully examine your biosketch—so an article under review isn't as good as an acceptance. If you have done good work, but have not published it, it may be wise to delay submission of a proposal for a cycle in order to get more articles out.

It is also useful to think about the types of articles you can write now. If you have done pilot work for a larger study that you are now proposing, you face a particular problem: You can describe the outcomes in your Preliminary Work section as soon as the study is complete, but you probably won't have time to publish these outcomes. You may have collected some preliminary findings on outcomes earlier as the study was ongoing. But let's be clear: You cannot publish some preliminary findings and then later publish the final findings. You can't say "Well here are our findings on the first 50 people in the study" and later on say "And here are our findings on the whole 100." If you publish on the first 50 participants, you cannot publish again on those participants. However, there are other relevant articles you can write and publish. For example, you can publish a review article in the area of your study: You will have reviewed the literature to make the case for the study; now you can refocus that review and turn it into a more general, state-of-the-science paper. (We have described the structure of a review paper in Chapter 4 on PhD proposals, and you may want to look at that chapter.) You may also have interesting baseline data on the people who took part in your pilot. For example, perhaps in your initial assessment you found that participants had little understanding of drug doses and great fear of drugs and this influenced their management of their disease. Or perhaps you have gained information about the challenges of working with a particular group like young African American men with hypertension, and you have developed strategies for engaging them. You could publish a paper on that topic. Or you conducted some focus groups with mothers of the adolescents in your study and found interesting ideas about what these women need—also a publishable paper. Or you have some ideas about recruitment and retention of a particular group of people. It is important to think broadly about what you can publish—but again, not to think about publishing preliminary results. That may be tempting but don't do it unless, like the old study of AZT efficacy in combating HIV infection, your preliminary results were so compelling that you stopped the study.

DEVELOPING A TEAM

While you are working on writing and publishing articles, focus also on putting together your team. Reviewers want to know that people on the team have the appropriate expertise and are the best people to do the project. First, think through what you plan to do, what those plans require, what your expertise is (which must be documented—you might be an expert in stroke rehabilitation but if your biosketch doesn't show that expertise, no one will believe in it), and what other expertise you need. If you are using smart phones to deliver an intervention, you probably need an expert in this technology on the team. If you are doing a qualitative study, either your biosketch needs to show some expertise in qualitative methods (through publications) or you need a co-investigator whose biosketch shows expertise in these methods. If you are planning to test an intervention to improve adherence to a low-sodium diet, you need someone in the team who is expert in improving adherence. If you are looking at health literacy, you need someone who understands it and knows how to measure it. If you are doing any statistical analyses, you must have a biostatistician or statistician on the team, even if you know how to do all the analyses (because the biostatistician's biosketch will show experience in analyzing data for funded studies, but yours won't).

Finding this expertise is more of a problem for researchers in small universities than for those in big, research-intensive universities with medical centers, but it is a challenge for new researchers anywhere. Think through your needs and contact people in your university who can provide the expertise you need in addition to your own. It is best to find your co-investigators in your university, both because that makes it easier to work together and because including co-investigators from outside requires a subcontract. However, if you can't find all the expertise you need in your university, look outside. If your study will be small with a miniscule budget, you will not be able to afford to pay co-investigators, but there may be people in your university who are expert in areas of your study and would be happy to work with you in exchange for the experience and co-authorships. You may be able to get "in-kind" (i.e., not paid) assistance from your school's statistician. And your budget may be able to support hiring a consultant who is an expert in your area and can guide you in the work. Figure out what you most need and think about how to get it.

You may want co-investigators to write something in their area (e.g., on recruitment methods or adaptation of the intervention for advanced technology), and if so, be sure to ask them about doing it before you put them on the team. Also, make sure the people you put on the team are going to work. There is never enough money to pay people just for their names.

One other thing—you need to show that your team is a team, not just an assemblage of unconnected people. The best way to show that is to have publications together. So when you are putting together publications, make sure you include team members in the writing.

Also, think about finding consultants to round out your expertise. They can come from anywhere; they don't require a subcontract, and their contributions are not expected to be huge. Their role is to ensure that you are on the right track in the areas they know about and you may not know about. Many experts in a variety of fields are extremely generous about serving as consultants, and you should not hesitate to ask those people to help you. (All they can do is say no.) However, if you ask an expert to consult on your grant, be sure to offer co-authorship on major publications to come from the work. And along those lines, it is helpful to discuss authorship and specifically first authorship with the team early on, so there are no misunderstandings later. Generally, if you are the principal investigator (PI), you should be first author on the major publications from the study; but others need first authorships, too, so think of other papers from the study that they can lead.

As you contact people for your team, remind them that you will need a biosketch from each of them. You want to make sure that all team members have a clear idea of the aims and methods of the study before they write these, and it is wise to check the biosketches before you submit the proposal to be sure that the personal statements people write are appropriate. They could sound like the authors don't know what the study is about, or they could sound like the author ought to be the PI. You don't want either of those.

If you are writing a PhD proposal or a DNP capstone project, you are on your own. There's no team of co-investigators to work with you. But you can get help and guidance from your committee. Before you begin, think about the best person to chair the committee: That person can be a great help to you (or not). From your courses, you probably have a good idea about who is a great chair; also ask others who are ahead of you in the process. And once you have a chair, figure out, with that person's help, what other expertise you will need, then look for committee members with the expertise.

FINDING SETTINGS

Next you need to figure out where you are going to conduct the study. This is a crucial question that you must answer early on, or you have no study. For example, if you plan to conduct a study in schools, you must figure out what permissions you need. Generally you must have permission from the school superintendent and principals of the particular schools where you recruit subjects. But you may also need permission from the school nurse. If you plan to conduct a study in a health department, whose permission do you need? The director? Clinical directors? What about a hospital unit? How far up the chain of command do you need to go? There are many horror stories of researchers who could not get permission to do their study; you don't want to contribute another one. This is particularly important for evidence-based practice projects: If you do not have buy-in from staff, champions to support you, and administrative backing, your project may never get off the ground. The key is to deal with this issue early, then, if you are doing research and you find that one setting will not work, you have time to find another. Or if you are planning an evidence-based practice project and you cannot gain the approvals you need, you can propose a different topic that staff and administrators may think more useful to the hospital or clinic.

If you plan to work in the community, it is very important to make some contacts with those in charge before you try to get their permission to conduct a study. For example, if you are interested in conducting a study in African American churches, it would be wise to build relationships with pastors of those churches before proposing to recruit their congregations.

It is also important to determine whether they have a health ministry and who is in charge, or what other groups in the church would be important to work with. And think about contributing something to the agency or community; don't just use the people.

Remember that you will need a letter of support from every site you plan to use. But don't ask the people in charge to write the letter; write a draft for them—don't call it a draft, say it's a brief summary of the study for them, and then they will put it on letterhead and sign. If you are using more than one site, do be sure to write different letters—don't make it obvious that the people signing are not the people writing.

WRITING THE PROPOSAL

Finding Time to Write

Clearly there are numerous logistical issues you need to deal with in preparing to submit a proposal. But don't forget that the major task is writing the proposal. To begin, think about the kind of time you will need to write. Some writers work in brief stints, a half hour or an hour, then they are done for the day. But many writers need a large block of time in which to write—and a little warm-up time, otherwise known as procrastination. However, this is productive procrastination—like pencil sharpening time. To get ready to write, people do mindless tasks like responding to e-mails or washing the car or cleaning the house or doing laundry in order to empty their minds of anything that would interfere with the intense concentration required for writing. Then they write. If you are this kind of writer, just make sure to allocate both enough time to warm up and to write, or you will have great laundry and a beautiful car but no proposal.

Once you have decided what kind of time you need, you must find a way to get that time. If you are lucky, you may get a buy out of one course you teach in order to spend time writing a proposal. But you may not be lucky. So you will have to make the time yourself. Here's one way to do that. Everyone needs to waste some time, but most of us waste more than we need to. Look at how you spend your days and you may find that you could waste 15 minutes less each day and save that time for writing. Also, when you look at your days, see if you can find ways to keep other people from wasting so much of your time. Probably you could save another 15 minutes a day that way. Taken together, that would amount to $2\frac{1}{2}$ hours a week. That's a good chunk of time.

If you work best for a half hour or hour, you should think about starting your day with writing. Put aside time before you go to the office or start writing in the office, with your door locked and before you open your e-mails. If you need a large block of time, figure out which days of the week are best for writing and mark off the time. If you are teaching, don't plan to work on your proposal on the day after an exhausting clinical; that is generally a recovery day. You want to write when you are at your sharpest, so think about the day before clinical, or a day when you are not obsessing about class preparation. Once you mark off the time, don't give it up, or you'll never get this done.

Then find a quiet spot—the office if you won't be interrupted, or home if you don't have small children who want you, or a library if need be. Sit down and begin. First make files for all the parts of the proposal specified in the funding agency's guidelines. For example, for the NIH, make files for Specific Aims, Significance, Innovation, Approach, and under Approach, put preliminary studies, design, setting, sample, intervention, variables and their measurement, and so forth. Get a notebook that you carry with you everywhere you go. Whenever you have a thought about one of these sections, write it down—these thoughts are likely to be important, but if you don't write them down, you'll forget them. And as you become engaged in writing this proposal, you find that you have ideas all the time—driving home, in the shower, at a cocktail party, not just when you are sitting in front of the computer. That is because when you are deeply engaged in any project, your head works on it round the clock, throwing up insights when least expected. Make sure you capture those. And as you work on the sections of the proposal, you may want to move back and forth—for example, you may find that you are stymied in trying to make the case for the study but you have concrete ideas for Methods. So switch to Methods. Then go back to that other section later.

Developing Purpose and Aims

When you are sitting at the computer, begin by sketching out your purpose and some aims; these are your first concern. Without them, you can have no sense of what you want to do or why, and no idea of how to do it. Begin with your general purpose. Will you test the feasibility of some intervention to improve the adoption process for prospective parents and children and collect initial data on its efficacy? What kind of intervention will you try? What specifically will you look at to determine feasibility or to indicate efficacy if that is an aim? Will you test hypotheses about the effects of the environment on the development of obesity in children? What aspects of the environment do you expect to be influential? How might you measure them?

Once you have a purpose that seems reasonable, write down some specific aims; that is, aspects of the overall purpose that are smaller but more precise and for which you can measure achievement. For example, if your overall purpose is to improve diabetes management among Hispanic women, your aims might be to increase their physical activity, improve their diet, increase their monitoring of blood glucose, and so forth. However, expect these aims to change as you refine your rationale for the study and your purpose and proposed methods. Your budget will also affect your aims; with small grants you can only do so much for so many. And with a dissertation or DNP proposal, you had best limit your aims to things you can actually do in the next year.

Developing the Rationale for the Study

Your next task is to develop the rationale for the study. You should already have a grasp of the literature: That's how you knew that something more needed to be done and how you developed the idea for a study in the first place. Now you want to go back to the literature or to your notes on the literature, and synthesize these to make the case for your proposed work—show its significance and innovation. You also need to recheck the databases to be sure nothing has been published since the last time you looked. Once you have a good idea of the rationale for your study, write a draft of the Significance section, or the Background section or Background and Significance section if that's what the funding agency calls it. We have suggested an approach to writing about the significance of the study in Chapter 2. It is important to produce a draft of this section early on since it affects everything else you write. Don't write this section to space specifications to begin with. Write what you think needs to be said and then cut back later on, when your sense of what you want to do is better developed. Finally, state your purpose again.

Next, if you have a conceptual framework, describe it and do a preliminary drawing of the framework. (Note that basic science proposals and more physiological proposals do not generally include a conceptual framework.) Then, if you are writing for the NIH, take a first stab at Innovation. In basic science proposals, this section is not hard to write, because it is obvious what is new about your approach. But in more clinical or behavioral proposals, this is often the hardest part to write. However, writing it helps you think about what is really new about your study—and helps you get rid of fluff. If you are not writing for the NIH, you probably do not have a separate section on innovation but talk about what is new in your study toward the end of the Significance or Background and Significance section.

Writing About Methods

You need to begin developing your methods in detail as you are writing the section on the rationale for the study. Reexamination of the literature may help with this: The studies you examine may give you clearer ideas about both your aims and ways to achieve them. For example, you may find that some of what you plan to do to prevent risky sex behaviors in adolescents has already been done, or recent research suggests better ways to intervene with mothers or fathers to help them help their adolescents, or technological developments suggest a more effective way to engage adolescents. With new information, your aims may change. Then your methods change.

Also, as you think about methods, you may discover that others have tried what you want to try and have found that it is not doable, or you may realize that your aims as currently stated are so fuzzy you can't figure out what to do; or you may find there's a better way to do something than you initially thought. And you may also realize that there will not be enough money in the grant you are seeking to do what you would like, or not enough time in your life to collect data from all those families you were targeting, so you need to scale back. This thinking affects your aims, and revised aims affect methods and so on. Indeed, as you move forward, you discover that anything you do affects nearly everything else you plan. Nothing is written in stone until far later in the process. This is especially true now that we tend to write on computers: Everything can be changed or deleted, so it doesn't feel as permanent as paper.

We have made numerous suggestions for developing your methods, both in the chapter on basic methods (Chapter 3) and in the chapter on NIH proposals (Chapter 5). Look at every reasonable option and keep notes about them; and keep a record of what you have planned and what you have jettisoned. You may want to return to some idea you abandoned earlier. Also, when you note in the proposal that you will do X even though Y looks feasible, you will need to justify that—and if you have good notes, you will be able to describe your reasoning.

As you write methods, make a subheading for everything in that section: Overview, Setting, Sample, Intervention (if applicable), Variables and Their Measurement, Procedures (if you include this section) and Data Management and Analysis. This helps you think about the methods. Fill in each section whenever you have a new thought.

DEVELOPING THE BUDGET AND OTHER MATERIALS

You also need to develop your budget and its justification now. Work with your budget office, but be clear about what you need to do and when so they can help you. We have made numerous suggestions for developing the budget in Chapter 12, and we recommend that you use those. Also, collect copies of your instruments for the Appendix, and make sure you have up-to-date biosketches from all members of the research team, letters of support from the sites you will be using, and a description of facilities and resources available to you.

REVISING THE PROPOSAL

Once you have a beginning draft of the rationale for your study and the methods you will use to carry it out, look at the two together and see if they match; if not, change one or the other and finish the first draft of the proposal. The first draft is the hardest to write—because you are trying to present your ideas and information in a logical fashion even though the mind doesn't generally work that way but tends to operate more circuitously, throwing up ideas about this and that but not presenting them in a linear fashion. It is hard to put those ideas together in a straight logical line. That's why this draft is so hard to write. However, the first draft is also the most exciting to write, because writing is not just reporting, it is discovery. When we write, we find that we know more than we thought we knew and we see things from new perspectives and discover relationships that we had never thought of before. Indeed, most people like writing (even if they hate beginning to write) because they discover new things as they write. And this produces a great euphoria. However, when we finish a first draft of anything—report, article, proposal, anything we have created—the experience of euphoria tends to rub off onto what we have written. So we think the draft is great; but in fact, most first drafts are incoherent at best.

Therefore, when you have finished your first draft, step away from your desk for a couple of days. Don't show the draft to anybody, don't even consider that. In order to see the draft as it is, you need to disconnect from it, so that you are not so much involved with it and your euphoria. Come back to the draft in a day or so and see what it looks like. Even a day away will give you some disconnect and enable you to see what you have written rather than what you hoped to write. Once you can begin to see what is actually on paper, you can make it better.

Print out your draft proposal, double spaced, and look at it; you see it better if it is in hard copy than on the computer screen, and you need a double-spaced version so you can write suggestions and edits on it. Your task now is to produce a coherent proposal. Remember that you are writing for reviewers, not for yourself, and you must help other people understand why your work needs to be funded. You can't assume that because you think it matters, others will also. Go through the proposal, looking first at your rationale for doing the study. If you are not sure it is compelling, you might try outlining the points to see if they make sense and add up to an argument. Look particularly at whether you have provided evidence of importance of the problem, adequately described the work already done on the problem, and, finally, shown why something more is needed. If you see a lot of irrelevant or peripheral information, delete it even though you hate doing that (but always keep a copy of what you have deleted in case you need to put it back in). If you aren't clear about the argument for the study, look back at our chapter on developing the rationale for a study and see if you have followed the suggested outline and included the important materials.

Next look at your purpose and aims, then at any hypotheses or research questions, and compare these to your methods. Do they fit? Do your methods show that you have the data to test the hypotheses? Have you provided a power analysis that shows you have a big enough sample for hypothesis testing? For many small studies or exploratory studies, you will not have a big enough sample to test hypotheses, so you may need to delete these. Sometimes people get around this problem by talking about "working hypotheses," which are essentially expectations that can't be tested in the proposed study. You can try that, or simply say "We expect that people who receive the intervention will show more improvement than those in a control group." Or you can use research questions.

Now look at your conceptual framework, if you included one. Does it show causes and consequences? Is it linear, or is it confusingly circular? And does the figure representing the framework reflect the description of it in the text? And finally, does this framework fit with what you are actually going to do?

Now look at your preliminary work. Have you described the team in such a way that together, you appear likely to succeed in conducting the study? Saying this is a great team is not enough; you have to show, not tell. And what about your description of preliminary work leading to the proposed study? Is it clear and coherent, showing purpose, methods, findings, and conclusions? Is the relationship of this work to the proposed study obvious?

Finally, go through your Methods section with a fine-toothed comb to see whether there are gaps or problems or illogic. Have you clearly described your proposed settings? Are the sample criteria reasonable? Have you shown that you can get enough participants who meet those criteria in those settings? Is your intervention (if you have one) presented in such a way that reviewers will be convinced that it can be done, it is likely to be efficacious, and it will be translatable to the real world of practice? Have you clearly described a comparison or control group? Are your data collection methods clear, and will reviewers understand the instruments you are using to collect data? Will those instruments tell us whether the intervention or experiment works? And what about your analyses: Are they appropriate, clearly described, and without extra padding? (It is important to make sure that a statistician or biostatistician is working with you to ensure that the analysis is appropriate and clear.) Finally, if you have decided to use particular methods when other available methods looked as good or better, make sure that you have presented your rationale for your decisions.

As you go through all of these sections, remember that the job now is to turn your rough first draft into a clear, coherent, and complete proposal that provides the reviewers all the information they need, in the order in which they need it, and nothing else. As you work through the draft, look everywhere for incoherence. For example, are you saying the same thing over and over again? Readers don't need to read most things but once, so if you see something on page 5 that sounds faintly familiar, look back and see whether you've already said it, and if so, decide where to put it: one place or the other, not both. Also, are you telling readers things they don't need to know? For example, do readers need to know that your team will meet on Wednesdays to go over study progress? No, what they want to know is that you will meet weekly, not what day, or what time.

Also make sure that you have put things in the right order. Setting comes before sample: Reviewers first want to know whether your setting is going to provide enough people to make up your sample; only then will they be interested in your specific criteria for including people in the sample. And the intervention comes before data collection: Reviewers want to know what you are going to do for people before you tell them what data you will collect to test that intervention's efficacy. And readers want some explanation of instruments before you tell them about the validity and reliability of those instruments. So think about the reader as you revise: What does the reader need, in what order, to follow your reasoning and be convinced that your study should be done?

Finally, make sure that you are clear about your logic. Writers sometimes stop explaining what they are thinking, though they don't stop thinking. Essentially they go underground for a time, then come up and make a point that seems to have nothing to do with what they said before. This is called a logical leap; but usually it is only the poor reader who has to make a leap. The writer is just silently thinking. But this silence can cost you. So always check your logic to be sure that you have not left out some of the links. Reviewers must see every step in your thinking.

Once you have a draft that seems coherent, print out the new draft both double spaced and single spaced. You want to keep working on the double spaced version, and you should use the single spaced version to see whether you are over the page limit and if so, by how much, and therefore see how much you need to cut. Now, go back and look at every sentence you have written to be sure that it says what you want to say, not gobbledygook. Remember that you are not trying to win a prize for complicated sentences but to convince reviewers that your study holds great promise and should be funded. Remember also that some of the people who review your study are not experts in your particular area, so you need not speak in shorthand. Rather, you want to write for intelligent readers. It is often helpful to read your sentences aloud to see whether they are clear: It can be a mortifying experience but it will help your prose.

When you are checking your sentences, it is particularly important to be clear about your conceptualizations: You may have discovered a theory that seems exciting to you, but it needs to be clear to readers, and its relevance to your work must be obvious. And you must be clear about definitions and distinctions: How are you defining depression? Depressive symptoms? The consequences of depression? If you are looking at the importance of religion and spirituality for disease management, how are you defining them? Are they separate? Do they overlap? If your definitions are fuzzy or shifting, this can cause unnecessary hostility on the part of reviewers—and you don't want that.

REVIEWS AND FURTHER REVISIONS

The next step is to get everyone on your team to read and comment on the proposal. Don't send the proposal to them unannounced: Let them know when it is coming and ask for a reasonable turnaround time to get comments. Take their suggestions for improvement and do another draft. But be careful that you are not being sent in the wrong direction. Then get some external reviewers to check the proposal. However, never send your proposal to external reviewers until you think you have done the absolute best you can, or you will waste their time and yours (and your money, external reviews don't come for nothing). Pick external reviewers who know the area and know what the NIH or the agency you are going to expects, and ask them in advance if they will review the proposal: Don't just send it out of the blue. Also, listen to their suggestions. You may do an internal mock review as well: Work with your research or facilitation office to set this up. It is often helpful to tape a mock review session to be sure you don't forget the suggestions. Again, listen to those suggestions. The problems that do writers in are never the problems they see: They are the problems writers don't see. In many cases, the mock reviewers or external reviewers show you problems that you have not seen, and if you don't deal with them, you are unlikely to get funded. It's easy to say, "They just don't understand"— but the fact is that they don't understand because you have not been clear. They are pointing to real problems. This is the time to listen, think, rethink, and revise accordingly.

After all the reviews and after you have made the revisions suggested, go back through the proposal once more to make sure that you are consistent throughout and everything matches and makes sense. Don't say you have a sample of 50 on page 8 and a sample of 150 on page 12. Make sure aims and methods are not contradictory, and cut out everything extra so that you fit within page limits. If you are over the page limits, first cut the peripheral information and then try to shorten your descriptions of what is essential; that's probably going to be easier to do in Significance than in Methods because you can probably cut or condense some of the description of work already done, but it's hard to cut methods at this point.

Here are a few tricks of the trade that help: Look at every paragraph that ends with half a line or less and see if you can cut enough words to gain a line. Use small words instead of big words, for example, "use" not "utilize," "in" not "within," and get rid of extra uses of "the" and extra phrases. Eventually you can make the proposal fit within the limits. If your proposal is complete but shorter than the allowed page length, reviewers will love you. However, if it is shorter, read it again and again to be sure you have included absolutely everything that is needed.

As you move toward a final draft, there is one thing to pay close attention to: If your PhD or DNP advisor or a funding agency gives you specific rules about preparing a proposal, follow them. For example, the NIH wants your proposal to be single spaced with margins that can be as small as .5 inches. So many people write and write and write and fill up all the space. But longer is not necessarily better. When the proposals go out to reviewers, the groans can be heard across the nation. Take our suggestions and edit to make sure your proposal is concise. Use tables and figures if they can help you summarize a lot of information in a shorter space (but don't just stick them in; always talk about them in the text). And leave as much white space as possible, perhaps an extra line between sections or paragraphs. And, remember, single spacing means just that. Choose single spacing in your word processing software. Six lines per inch, not eight lines per inch, not 1.15 line spacing. Single spacing. If the institution or agency to which you are applying asks for double spacing, then double space. But don't try to cheat. Your proposal, and all of your work, may be disqualified on a technicality.

If you have someone helping you prepare the final proposal, help them help you! Make sure the person has a copy of the guidelines for the proposal, what font is required, what font size is required, what margins and page lengths are allowed, and so forth. Finally, give the proposal to the grants or research office for preparation and submission, along with a cover letter saying where you'd like the proposal to go, if at the NIH. And stay around to assist with any last minute details: You are ultimately responsible for the quality and completeness of the final product.

FIFTEEN

SUBMISSION AND REVIEW OF THE PROPOSAL

SUBMISSION

If you are submitting a proposal to your dissertation committee or capstone project committee, be sure to follow the guidelines that your school and your chair provide. For example, make sure to give committee members enough time to read your proposal—often 2 weeks are required. You may need to meet with each of them before the defense of your proposal to get their input and suggested proposal revisions; also, some students are required to have an oral defense of their proposal for the committee, so if this is true for you, you will want to prepare your defense presentation in advance and be sure to observe the time specifications that you are provided.

Funders often have detailed requirements about how proposals are to be submitted. They may require a paper submission or an electronic submission. They may have a "mailed by" or a "received by" due date. They may allow exceptions for natural disasters, or they may not. They may or may not require cover letters (but you should always provide one). In any event, you and your institution need to know the rules and follow them to the "t." You do not want all of your hard work to be for naught.

Federal agencies have very explicit guidelines. For example, the National Institutes of Health (NIH) proposals are usually to be submitted electronically by the institution—generally, you do not submit the proposal yourself, your institution does it for you since awards are typically made to them. But if the institution waits until the last minute to submit the proposal, the Internet could be "busy" or "down" or you might have errors in the proposal that could have been corrected if only you had had time. The NIH used to have an "error correction window" that enabled you to respond to errors and warnings that their software identified, but this window has been eliminated, so be sure to have the proposal submitted earlier than the deadline in case you need to make corrections. Please note, however, that the software does not check the content of what you have written in the proposal—that is up to you. So check the final proposal to be sure it says what you want it to—do not rewrite it at this point, just check it!

Approvals—Get Them!

When your institution submits the proposal electronically for you, it is the same as if it has "signed off" on a paper version of the proposal, guaranteeing that it meets their expectations and that certain assurances are provided and policies are in place (e.g., misconduct in science, conflict of interest, age and sexual discrimination, civil rights). They are likely to check certain portions of your proposal very carefully (e.g., the budget, promises you have made on their behalf), and they usually require that you or your school acquire appropriate signatures from within the institution. Often these include signatures from the leader of your school as well as those of the schools of other investigators on the research team.

Make sure to allow sufficient time for this process. The various schools that need to sign off may require time to have someone read the proposal, review the budget for their particular individuals, or perhaps even negotiate a share of the facilities and administration (F&A; indirect costs; overhead) that your school will be getting. The larger institution (the university or clinical agency) requires time to perform its review, get feedback from you if there are questions, and submit the proposal. So be sure to ask how much time is needed for each of these approval steps, put them on your calendar, and follow them. (Sometimes you can submit things such as the budget to the approvers while you are still working on the guts of the proposal; if you find yourself needing to do this, ask instead of assuming that it will be okay.)

Cover Letter

The NIH now requires a cover letter attachment for most proposals; the SF424 (R&R) even tells you what to put in the letter and how to format it. Among other things, they want to know to which of their institutes you are requesting assignment for possible funding, which group(s) you wish to review the proposal and which you do not, what disciplines are involved in the proposal (if it is multidisciplinary), and so on. Thus, read the guidelines carefully and do as they request. But know that, ultimately, the NIH will make the decisions about where your proposal goes for review and possible funding. Other agencies may also require a cover letter; check their guidelines.

REVIEW

When you submit a proposal, one or more people are going to review what you have written. This may be a series of sequential reviews to determine whether you are qualified to submit the proposal, whether it is on a topic that is relevant for the agency, whether you have submitted all the required sections, and what the merit of the proposal is. Sometimes your proposal will get kicked out of the system before it has even made it to review. Therefore, we encourage you to speak with the agency prior to going through all the work of preparing a proposal. You want to be sure they are interested in what you are proposing before you get all the way to the review.

When the science of the proposal is reviewed, you hope that the reviewers will provide you with their feedback, but unfortunately this is not always the case. PhD and Doctor of Nursing Practice (DNP) committee members will provide you with feedback so you can learn from their input and revise the proposal and your approach to the project. Foundations and small-grant funders sometimes provide feedback and sometimes do not; Health Resources and Services Administration (HRSA) provides some feedback, whereas the NIH provides rather extensive reviews. The NIH model, described later, shows clearly what happens to your proposal once it is submitted.

Receipt and Assignment of the Proposal

At the NIH, proposals are submitted to the Center for Scientific Review (CSR), one of the institutes and centers at the NIH, and individuals there use things such as the cover letter with your requests, the funding opportunity announcement (FOA) to which you are responding, the proposal, and the investigators' backgrounds and expertise to decide what institutes or centers might be right for funding the project and where to send it for review. Note that while two institutes or centers may be identified for possible funding of your proposal (and ultimately, they may decide to share that funding), such "dual assignment" does not come with dual review—only one review will be conducted of your proposal even if it is dually assigned for possible funding. Some FOAs are quite clear that the review will occur under the auspices of an institute, in which case your proposal will be assigned to that institute for review and possible funding. In other cases, one of the many review groups at the CSR may be assigned to do the review, and an institute will be selected as a possible funder.

The CSR assigns your proposal a number that is composed of a type, activity code, one or two funding institute(s) code(s), serial number, and grant year, and indicating whether or not the proposal is an amendment (revision) to a prior submission or possibly a supplemental request. The principal investigator(s) (PIs) are informed about the decisions the CSR has made about the proposal via the electronic Research Administration (eRA) Commons, which is how the NIH communicates with you (they currently also use e-mail, but that may go by the wayside in the future), so be sure to have the appropriate individual in your home institution sign you up well in advance of the submission and include your eRA Commons user name where requested in the application and on the biosketch. Then, check the site frequently after your proposal has been submitted so you stay up-to-date on all developments. If you disagree with any of the assignment decisions, contact the CSR right away so you can make your preferences known.

Informing the Possible Funder

We also recommend that when you submit a proposal to the NIH, you inform the program director at the institute or center with whom you have been speaking. Let them know that your proposal has been submitted, but also send the person a few key pieces of information: at least send them the PI name (this may not be as obvious as it sounds—they may know you by a nickname, but your proposal may be submitted using your formal, full name), the final title of the proposal, and the abstract. You may also wish to send the Specific Aims section if that adds anything to what you have said in the abstract. At a minimum, you want to thank the person for the help given you, and if you and the person agree that the proposal would find a good home in her or his institute or center, perhaps she or he can be on the lookout for the proposal and help get it assigned to that institute or center.

The Review: Who, How, and When?

At the NIH, most standing study sections at the CSR meet three times per year; however, if your proposal will be reviewed by an initial review group in an institute or by a special emphasis panel that has been established just for these proposals, the meetings may be held only once, or once a year. Typically, there are about 20 reviewers at a meeting, with phone and written reviews also coming into the mix. Who are these people? Usually, they are scientists like you—but typically they are people who have been funded to do their research, have published their findings, and have achieved a certain level of success. (You can learn who these people are through your eRA Commons account once you have submitted or via the NIH webpage of the CSR or the institute that is reviewing your proposal.) You may find that the NIH is using newer scientists in their reviews, so be on the lookout for review opportunities in your area—just do not spend all

TABLE 15.1 Review Criteria for Selected NIH Proposals

	Research and Research Center (R, DP, RC, P, etc.)	AREA (R15)	Fellowship (F30, F31, F32, F33)	Career Development (K01, K02, K07, K08, K23, K24, K25, K99)
Overall Impact	Overall Impact	Overall Impact	Overall Impact/Merit	Overall Impact
Scored Review Criteria (Scored individually and considered in overall impact score) PAR and RFA: May add questions to each scored criterion or additional criteria	✓ Significance ✓ Investigator(s) ✓ Innovation ✓ Approach ✓ Environment	✓ Significance ✓ Investigator(s) ✓ Innovation ✓ Approach ✓ Environment	✓ Fellowship Applicant ✓ Sponsors, Collaborators, and Consultants ✓ Research Training Plan ✓ Training Potential ✓ Institutional Environment and Commitment to Training	✓ Candidate ✓ Career Development Plan/Career Goals and Objectives/Plan to Provide Mentoring ✓ Research Plan ✓ Mentor(s), Co-Mentor(s), Consultant(s), Collaborator(s) ✓ Environment and Institutional Commitment to the Candidate
Additional Review Criteria (Not scored individually, but considered in overall impact score) PAR and RFA: May add questions to each criterion or additional criteria	R01 -BRP only: • Partnership and Leadership All: ✓ Protections for Human Subjects	✓ Protections for Human Subjects ✓ Inclusion of Women, Minorities, and Children ✓ Vertebrate Animals ✓ Biohazards • Resubmission • Renewal • Revision	✓ Protections for Human Subjects ✓ Inclusion of Women, Minorities, and Children ✓ Vertebrate Animals ✓ Biohazards • Resubmission • Renewal	✓ Protections for Human Subjects ✓ Inclusion of Women, Minorities, and Children ✓ Vertebrate Animals ✓ Biohazards • Resubmission • Renewal • Revision
Additional Review Considerations (Not scored individually and not considered in overall score)		• Select Agents • Resource Sharing Plans ✓ Budget and Period of Support	✓ Training in the Responsible Conduct of Research • Applications From Foreign Organizations • Select Agents • Resource Sharing Plans ✓ Budget and Period of Support	✓ Training in the Responsible Conduct of Research • Select Agents • Resource Sharing Plans ✓ Budget and Period of Support
Additional Comments to Applicant		Additional Comments to Applicant	Additional Comments to Applicant	Additional Comments to Applicant

From the NIH (2014).

your time reviewing others. It takes a lot of time, and you want to develop your own scientific credentials.

Three to five reviewers are usually assigned to review your proposal in detail, with one or more serving as the primary, secondary, and tertiary reviewer(s). These individuals review the proposal in advance of the meeting using the review criteria discussed in earlier chapters and summarized here in Table 15.1 (also found at www.grants.nih.gov/grants/peer/Review_Criteria_at_a_Glance_MasterOA.pdf and using critique templates that can be found at www.public.csr.nih.gov/ReviewerResources/SpecificReview Guidelines/Pages/default.aspx). In addition to the main "scored" review criteria, each type of proposal has additional review criteria, considerations, and comments.

Each reviewer assigns scores ranging from 1 to 9 for each of the scored criteria and provides a similar 1 to 9 rating for the overall impact of the application (Table 15.2). Overall impact takes into account the scored criteria but is not meant to be an average of those scores; instead, it reflects the impact that the proposed work will have on the field *given* the criteria that are considered.

Reviews are submitted electronically to the NIH in advance of the review meeting so that preliminary average impact scores can be calculated and reviewers can see others' reviews of the proposals they have reviewed. Proposals are rank ordered based on their average impact scores, and those in the bottom half of the rankings usually are not discussed (i.e., are triaged out) so reviewers can spend their time discussing the more promising

TABLE 15.2 NIH Individual Scoring System for Each Scored Criterion and the Overall Impact Score

Overall Impact or Criterion Strength	Score	Descriptor
High	1	Exceptional
	2	Outstanding
	3	Excellent
Medium	4	Very Good
	5	Good
	6	Satisfactory
Low	7	Fair
	8	Marginal
	9	Poor

From the NIH (2013).

proposals (note, however, that reviewers can ask that a proposal be moved out of the triaged group if they wish to discuss it). At the meeting, the three to five reviewers assigned to the proposal are asked to indicate their "level of enthusiasm" (overall impact level) for the proposal. The primary reviewer presents the proposal and gives the major review points, and the secondary and tertiary reviewers add anything they wish. A general discussion of the proposal by all committee members ensues, and this is followed by a determination of the "level of enthusiasm" range, with original levels adjusted by the reviewers based on the various views expressed. Members eligible to vote then indicate their level of enthusiasm by giving each proposal an overall impact score in or near the specified range. After the meeting, these scores are averaged and the average is multiplied by 10, so that each discussed proposal ends up with a score between 10 and 90, with those closest to 10 being the best. (For proposals such as R01s, the NIH also gives applicants a percentile score that tells them where they stand in relation to other submissions during the current review cycle and, sometimes, up to two prior cycles.)

The CSR has a wealth of information available to applicants, including videos such as *NIH Peer Review Revealed*, so we encourage you to explore their website at www.public.csr.nih.gov/ApplicantResources/Pages/default.aspx. Just because you are an applicant (and thus will want to look at their offerings on "Applicant Resources"), do not ignore the "Reviewer Resources" links, because those have much to offer you as well. It is under the "Reviewer Resources" link that you will find the review criteria, scoring system and procedure, the difference between overall impact and significance, and so forth.

This review is not the only one that NIH conducts. In addition, each institute or center is advised by a National Advisory Council that will perform a second review of proposals that are being considered for funding. Typically, their goal is not to examine the science once again, but to advise the director about whether funding should be provided to your proposal. What if your proposal is strong scientifically but is not targeted at one of their priority areas? Should the institute consider it for funding? These are the types of things the National Advisory Councils consider.

If you are submitting somewhere other than the NIH, the review process is probably very similar, but it may be a little less formal: Proposals may be reviewed less frequently, the review panel may be larger or smaller, and the panel may be more broadly formed, with representatives from other entities such as professional practice or the community. The Patient-Centered Outcomes Research Institute (PCORI), for example, desires to fund proposals that improve patient-centered outcomes, so patients and other health care stakeholders are quite important to them.

Generally, reviews done by funders are expected to be confidential; reviewers are not to share the information about your proposal with others, and you are not to contact the reviewers. Any reviewer who has a conflict of interest with you or anyone on your investigative team should *not* participate in the review; different agencies handle such conflicts in different ways, but they all should require that the person in conflict exempt herself or himself from the review.

WAITING FOR THE FEEDBACK

Waiting for the feedback can be murder, but no matter to whom you are submitting your proposal, the review process takes time. If you are either hand or electronically delivering proposals to your committee members for a PhD or DNP degree, they will need time to read what you have prepared and may wish to speak with you about questions they have. If you are submitting to an agency such as the NIH, time is needed to assign your proposal to a review section and institute, see what proposals are in the mix, perhaps identify reviewers if they do not already have them on board, get the proposals to folks, give them time to do their reviews, allow them to submit their reviews, hold the review meeting, and write up the discussion that occurred at the meeting. The NIH receives (and reviews) over 80,000 proposals a year. That is a lot of reviewing. Therefore, the process can take weeks or months. Use this time productively, continuing to conduct current studies, analyze data, and write articles and submit them for publication. Also, if you have got the guts, reread the proposal and conduct a postmortem with your team, because you might see ways to strengthen the project or proposal should you need or wish to resubmit it. Also, you might want to stay on the lookout for other opportunities to submit the proposal. You will always need to tell an agency about other submissions you have made for the same project, but (a) that does not mean you cannot do so, and (b) you might want to consider revising the proposal into a slightly different project so both versions can be funded.

GETTING AND SURVIVING THE FEEDBACK

The NIH posts the scores to your eRA Commons account as quickly as it can. Typically, this is within 2 to 3 days of the end of the review meeting. But while the score is provided to you quickly, the review itself usually takes longer—often 4 to 6 weeks. (If you are a new investigator, this process can be and usually is faster, so you can consider revising and resubmitting more quickly should that be a step you need and wish to take.) Why does it take so long? Individual reviews have to be assembled and the discussion needs to be summarized (unless your proposal was triaged out and thus "not discussed," in which case you will receive the individual reviews but not a summary of the discussion, because there wasn't one). Note that the score and the reviews you receive are a private communication and are not visible to just every Tom, Dick, and Harry, but you are encouraged to share what you get—both score and reviews—with the rest of your team and anyone who advised or helped you with the preparation of the proposal.

If you get a perfect score (10), you can be pretty sure that you will be funded; congratulations! If you get a score that is not perfect (as the vast majority of us do), you will immediately start wondering what the problems were. You will dream up all sorts of stuff. You might want to contact the program officer to see if she or he can shed any light on what the score means. In most cases, the person cannot really tell you if the proposal will be funded, but she or he might be able to help clarify things if she or he or any colleagues attended the review meeting or listened to it electronically. Of course, they cannot add any insights if the proposal was not discussed, but even in these cases you will still receive the individual reviews, which can be *very* informative. How in the heck do you survive the uncertainty? Any way you can.

Some agencies provide little or no feedback from the review. You might get a letter or an e-mail that merely indicates that your proposal was or was not funded. Perhaps, there were lots of good proposals and they could not fund them all. These responses are hard to deal with, because you do not know whether there were specific issues with what you proposed or the agency just was not interested in the topic. You might want to try calling the program officer at the agency to see if you can get any additional information. Typically, you cannot, but you never know!

If you have submitted a PhD or DNP proposal, you might get lots and lots of feedback on the proposal, and you might get additional feedback as the proposal is discussed in your defense. Ask in advance whether you can record the defense so you do not have to take notes during the meeting, but if the answer is "no," you will want help writing down the suggestions, so you might want to ask the committee chair if she or he will help make sure that the major suggestions are noted. Make sure to gather up the drafts of the proposal with comments, and if a revision is required, use these drafts and the suggestions made at the meeting as guides. Many times, proposal reviews result in suggestions for conducting the project a bit differently, but you are not required to revise the proposal. In those cases, use the input to revise how you conduct the study, but also use it to guide how you write the final dissertation or capstone project report. Let's say you have three people on your committee; lay out those three versions side-by-side and go through them page by page. Suggested edits can be used to guide your preparation of the final document if you agree with them; if you do not agree with them, you may want to speak to the person who made them or to your chairperson to figure out a resolution. Where there are questions, you might need to make the presentation clearer, and where there are conflicts, discuss the issue(s) with your chairperson so resolutions can be reached.

REFERENCES

National Institutes of Health. (2013, March). Retrieved from https://grants.nih
.gov/grants/peer/guidelines_general/scoring_system_and_procedure.pdf
National Institutes of Health. (2014, March). Retrieved from https://grants.nih
.gov/grants/peer/Review_Criteria_at_a_Glance_MasterOA.pdf

SIXTEEN

NEXT STEPS

ANALYZING THE REVIEWS OF A PROPOSAL

If this was a PhD proposal or a Doctor of Nursing Practice (DNP) proposal, you have all the feedback in hand—maybe more than you will ever want. So move ahead on it. Unlike other proposal writers, you have the luxury of having your reviewers (committee members) nearby so you can ask them if you have questions about their comments. Consult with your chair if committee members' comments conflict and you are not sure how to proceed, but always respond to everything you can. And don't just ignore input from a committee member. If you choose not to make a requested change, explain why you made this decision in a side note or in person so she or he won't think you just ignored the input.

If your proposal was submitted for funding, you may or may not get feedback from the funding agency. If the proposal was submitted to the National Institutes of Health (NIH), however, you will get detailed critiques. So let us use the NIH proposal as a model for dealing with reviews. Once you receive the reviews, you will want to show them to and meet with your investigative team. You will want these individuals to have a copy of the reviews in their original state, but you will also want to use the information in the reviews to make a summary table or presentation of everything that was said. Remember that typically multiple people have reviewed your proposal, and multiple people have commented on the same sections, perhaps even making similar comments. Therefore, take what is in the reviews and re-present the information (a) organized by topic, (b) indicating which reviewer made the comment (or whether it was summarized in the discussion section), and (c) providing a space indicating your response to the comment. It might look like Table 16.1. Expand the table as needed to include what reviewers said in each section, but if nothing is said about a particular section, you can leave it out entirely. Some of the comments will be positive, and these are wonderfully helpful to your ego, but they do not need to take up much space in the table because the goal is to decide how you will respond to the criticisms raised.

Next, get the input of people who advised you during the proposal-writing process and even knowledgeable local people, if they might be of help to you. Perhaps there are people at your institution who review for the agency to which you submitted. Perhaps you have a grant-support office at your institution that might have helpful folks. In any event, use the people at your disposal. Give them the original reviews as well as your team's analysis of the reviews in advance of meeting with them so they have time

TABLE 16.1 Possible Format for Analyzing National Institutes of Health Research Reviews

Topic (Expand and Add Rows as Needed for Detailed Comments)	Reviewer/ Discussion	Response/ Plan to Resolve
Specific Aims		
Research Strategy Significance		
Innovation		
Approach		
Preliminary Studies		
Design		
Setting		
Sample		
Intervention		
Control/Comparison Group		
Variables and Their Measurement		
Procedures		
Plans for Data Analysis		
Timeline		
Human Subjects		
Budget and Justification		
Facilities and Other Resources		

to consider the issues. Remember, though, if you ask 10 people how to do something, you might get 10 different opinions. So the goal is to get the input and then have you and your team make the final decisions about whether and how to respond to the reviews.

DECIDING WHAT TO DO NEXT

Once you, your team, and any others you will be approaching have examined the reviews, you have a decision to make: If the proposal is not going to be funded, what is the appropriate next step? Is it to conduct more preliminary work? Publish? Revise the proposal and resubmit? Move on to other things? You do not want to waste the work you have done, but you also do not want to automatically resubmit. Make this decision with your team or mentors based on the overall tenor of the reviews, the score given by the study group (or the absence of an overall score), and the comments made by individual reviewers.

Some issues can be solved by writing more clearly and logically, or strengthening the case for the study's significance, or redesigning the study or analysis plans or adding new measures. You may also need to revise other sections, especially the Human Subjects or Vertebrate Animal sections. These changes are generally not that difficult to make. However, some reviewers want you to do more than revise the proposal. They want more preliminary work, or more publications of the work you have done, or more or different expertise on the study team.

Think about what the reviewers are asking for and decide whether you can do what they want, and then whether you want to do it. Never ignore the critiques: All reviewers will have a copy of those critiques and they will look carefully at whether you have responded to them. If you are not going to respond to the critiques with the changes needed, it is pointless to resubmit. You can't send a proposal back thinking, "Well, this time they'll get it." And you had best think twice (or more) about whether you want to make an argument for a study the reviewers did not like. Such arguments are not often successful.

So the first real question is, are you going to move forward or move on? If you decide to move forward, note that for resubmissions, the NIH requires a summary statement in electronic Research Administration (eRA) Commons, changes in the application, and a one-page introduction responding to issues raised in the reviews and summarizing the changes made. For proposals requiring letters of reference, you also need new letters.

RESUBMITTING THE PROPOSAL

Now begin the process of resubmission. Do not expect to do it in a day, and do not rush to resubmit. Whereas the NIH allows only one resubmission, they do allow 37 months from the time of the first submission for the resubmission. (Note that newer NIH rules allow you to submit a proposal again, as a new proposal, even if it has been turned down twice; but bear in mind that on "new" proposals you are not allowed to respond to the critique you received.) If the reviewers want more preliminary work, do that first. If you need funding to do more work, you can try for smaller funding from your university or a specialty organization or foundation, or you can step back from a major proposal like an R01 and apply to the NIH for more exploratory funding through an R03 or R21, or even an R15. Your timetable for resubmission will depend on completion of the additional preliminary work. Do not resubmit until you have the results of that work to guide what you plan to do.

If the reviewers want more publications, concentrate first on writing articles. And plan a timeline that will allow any additional preliminary work to be completed and the major article or articles to get accepted (i.e., be officially "in press") before you resubmit. Remember that only articles in press can be mentioned in most biosketches. And a frequent and damning critique is that the investigators have not published their work.

Now go through the table you made of the critiques and see what changes are needed. If the reviewers said that your conceptual framework was not adequately reflected by the study methods, or your conceptualization was not clear, you need to do some rethinking before you begin revising. It may help to outline the points in your framework and then compare these to the methods and outcomes you are proposing; if they do not match, change one or the other. If reviewers said your study would not have much of an impact, look at the Significance section and figure out how to make a stronger case for the importance of the proposed work. (Also, always go back to the literature to see whether new work has been done since your first submission, and include that.) If reviewers said your work was not innovative and would not add much to the science, look back at your Innovation section to see why and how it is weak and how you can strengthen it. For methodological problems, get help from an expert in study methods, and if the problem is your analysis, consult a statistician. If your proposal is for a career development award or fellowship, reviewers may have noted weaknesses in the training, so you need to strengthen your training plan, and perhaps find new mentors.

While you want to pay close attention to reviewers' critiques and address them as much as possible, reviewers are human like the rest of us and occasionally they are wrong. If you disagree with their suggestions, make the argument for the approach you have decided on in the introduction you write to the resubmission. For example, you could say that you have carefully considered the suggestions of reviewers but you have concluded that your approach will be more successful for the following reasons; then list them and make sure that the reasoning for that approach is clear.

Once you have thought through the major criticisms of the work and gotten a handle on the changes you need to make, go through your table of criticisms methodically and address each of them. If you have done more preliminary work, summarize that in the text. If you have had an article accepted, update your biosketch. (And update the biosketches of your team as well.) If you have added a new team member, make sure to say that in describing your team and preliminary work, and get a biosketch from that person. If you have added a booster session to the intervention, give reasons for it and describe it. If you have changed measurements or added some, describe them. If you have improved your analysis plans, make that clear. Finally, if reviewers noted problems that you cannot address or suggested approaches that you do not think are appropriate for your study, restate more clearly your plans and explain the reasoning behind the decisions you made.

When you have a more or less final draft of your revised proposal, write the introduction page—don't write it until you are clear about revisions, or you will have to rewrite it again and again as your plans change. The introduction is not really an introduction; it is a summary of your responses and the changes you have made in response to the reviewers' critiques. To begin, thank the reviewers for their careful critique of your review and note that you have made the changes suggested and this has strengthened your proposed work greatly. Don't waste precious space going on and on about how much you appreciate the fact that the earlier reviewers thought your work was really important. One sentence about how great they thought you were is enough. Remember that these current reviewers have a copy of the last review, so they know what was said.

It is best to go through the critiques by section of the proposal, not by reviewer, so as not to waste space repeating things that more than one reviewer said. However, in these sections, you may sometimes need to point out a particular reviewer's comments. Begin each section by briefly noting reviewers' issues (do that in a clause or phrase or you will waste precious space), then summarize your responses. For example, if reviewers were concerned about your conceptualization, briefly point out the clarifications you have made. If reviewers were concerned about the sample size, point out that you have increased the number of people you will recruit. If they were concerned about your analysis, note how you have refined it. Be sure to check what you say here against your revisions in the text to make sure that everything is consistent, and if space permits, you can refer reviewers to the appropriate sections of the text to find your changes.

Writers often feel some anger at reviewers: They did not understand what you were saying, or they did not realize that you had made things clear that they questioned. As you write your responses to reviewers, you will be tempted to express this anger at the critiques. For example, when a reviewer has said that you did not make X clear, but you think you did, it is tempting to say, "Reviewer *Y* thought we did not say *X*, but it was right there on page *Z*." Don't do that. Suppress your anger, and get someone else to read this page and check to make sure your anger is not coming out sideways. If a reviewer missed the point, say you have now clarified the point. You want to be infinitely polite and grateful for the help you have received from reviewers. Finally, check your introduction page once more against the proposal text and get ready to resubmit. It is helpful to have someone else also check the introduction against the text to be sure they match.

GETTING FUNDED OR APPROVED FOR IMPLEMENTATION

If you submitted your proposal to the NIH and you got a fundable score, the National Advisory Council will need to meet and a funding decision made before you find out whether your proposal might be selected for funding. Other agencies have their own procedures, but often there are multiple steps before funding can be awarded.

Getting "The Word"

How do you find out whether you are funded or approved for implementation? You need official word, not just your thinking that things are good to go. If you have applied for funding, you should receive an official Notice of Grant Award (NGA) that specifies the start date of the project. It should also indicate the end date, the amount of funding, and any rules for expenditure of those funds. For example, if you need to spend funds before the official start date, are you allowed to do so? Is the funding awarded to your institution or to you? If to you, are there tax consequences? Exactly how much money was awarded and in what categories? Can you move money between categories if needed or must it stay in the "pots" it is in? And so forth. The NGA should also specify any requirements there are if you accept the award: You certainly have to do the project, but does it have to be exactly as proposed? When are reports due to the funder? Can you extend beyond the end date of the project if needed? And so forth. Read the NGA very carefully and make sure to keep a copy with your project records; you will probably need to refer to it often. If you find anything that is questionable or of concern to you, get it resolved right away, in writing, before the project period starts. The biggest issue that usually arises is when the proposal proposes to do things one way, but reviewers suggested an alternative. Which do you do? Discuss this with the funder in advance of starting the project.

For those who are seeking funding from the NIH, the NGA comes to you via the eRA Commons. Other agencies may have similar mechanisms in place, or they may send you a letter or an e-mail.

Doing What You Said You Would Do

Whatever you are proposing to do, once approved or funded, *do what you said you would do.* If you are proposing to do a study of some sort, the first step is usually submitting a proposal to your local institutional review board (IRB) and getting it approved *before* you start to conduct the study. The exception to this is often in situations where you have a "delayed onset" of the study (e.g., due to training). In these cases, your first step may not be to obtain IRB approval, but it certainly needs to be done prior to the start of the study.

Hopefully, you designed a start-up period into your timeline, so during this time, you will want to make sure your team is ready to go, do everything you can to hire the necessary project personnel, set up space for them to work, get the settings fully on board (it has probably been a long time since you spoke with them at the proposal-writing stage), copy instruments if needed, and so forth. Use the time wisely for it seems to go by very quickly. Hit the ground running! Remember that the more quickly you hire your personnel, the more quickly you will have help! And once you begin, keep track of everything, recruit subjects, and carry out the study rigorously.

Reporting and Publishing

For those doing a PhD or DNP project, typically the "reporting" required involves regular meetings with your committee chair or advisor and then reporting the final outcomes via the dissertation or capstone project report. The form that document (or, in some cases, those documents!) take, depends on your institution, so you will want to have those details in hand well before you start.

For those who have obtained funding, some agencies only fund for short periods of time (e.g., 1 year or less) and only require a final report from you. Others, such as the NIH, require annual reports for most multi-year projects. There is a formal reporting format and certain things are required: Have you recruited the numbers of subjects, and particularly minorities, women and children, you said you would recruit? Are you following the methods you proposed? Are you in sync with the timeline you submitted? How are expenditures going with the budget? Basically, the funder is trying to learn how you are doing on all fronts. Be honest. Subjects tend to dry up the minute you start a study, so hopefully you did not overpromise in your proposal—hopefully you were realistic.

Finally, publish, publish, publish. No matter what type of project you are doing, you will want to share your discoveries with others. If you do not share them, the project will have been for naught. If you do, you may help to change the world.

INDEX

Printed in the United States
by Bookmasters

Printed in the United States
By Bookmasters